SIMPLE FOODS TO HEAL YOUR BODY

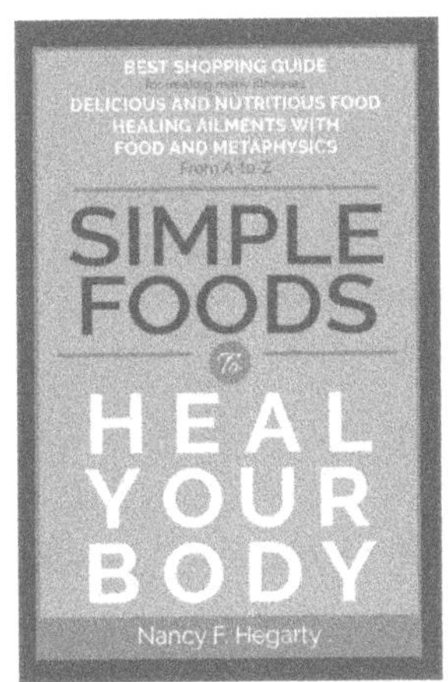

Nancy F. Hegarty

National Library Catalogue

Creator: Hegarty, Nancy F., author
Title: Simple foods to heal your body / Nancy F. Hegarty ; Laila Savolainen, illustrator.
ISBN: 9780992403478 (paperback)
ISBN: 9780992403447 (ebook)
Subjects: Natural foods.
Diet therapy.
Nutrition.
Other Creators/Contributors: Savolainen, Laila Kristina, 1967- illustrator.
Dewey Number: 641.302

Publisher
Paradise Waters Pty Ltd
P.O. Box 1856, Innisfail,
Queensland, Australia 4860

Disclaimer

The author of this book does not dispense medical advice nor prescribe the use of any technique as a form of treatment for medical problems without the advice of a health professional, either directly or indirectly. This book is not intended as a substitute for medical recommendations of healthcare providers. The intent is to offer information to help the reader co-operate with health professionals in a mutual request for optimum well-being.

Because any material can be misused, the author and publisher are not responsible for any adverse effects or consequences resulting from the use of any of the procedures suggested in this book. The author disclaims any liability in connection with the use of this information.

The publisher and author are not responsible for any goods and/or services offered or referred to in this book and expressly disclaim all liability in connection with the fulfilment of orders for any such goods and/or services and for any damage, loss or expense to the person or property arising out of or relating to them.

The publisher and author cannot accept responsibility for any mishap resulting from the use of any remedy described in this book. The ideas, procedures and suggestions contained in this book are not intended to replace the services of a trained health professional.

Dedication

I dedicate this book to all the beings on our beautiful planet. Each is gifted with a magnificent human body to love. May you be able to fill it daily with positive mood food, 'down to earth' goodness given by Mother Nature - to nurture and enjoy - food and heavenly rainwater.

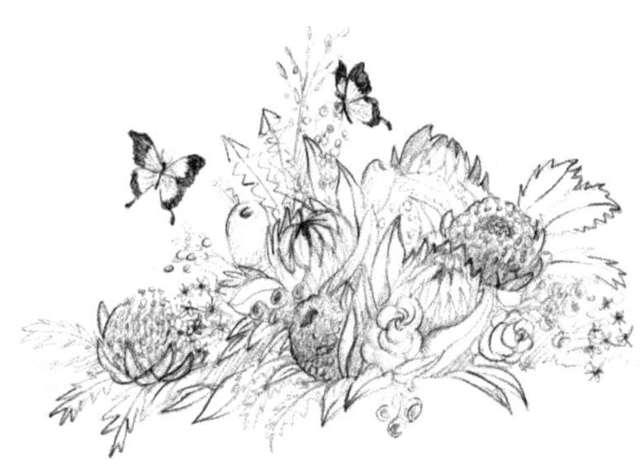

Nancy F. Hegarty

CDs

Daily Relaxation Meditation

Pain Management & Preparation for Healing (Meditation)

Meditation for Mustering Intensive Energy

An Introduction to a Healthy Life (positive affirmations to music with beats)

EBooks

The Australian Massage

Simple Foods to Heal Your Body

The Australian Advanced and Metaphysical Massage

BOOKS

The Australian Massage

Simple Foods to Heal Your Body

The Australian Advanced and Metaphysical Massage

DVD

The Australian Massage

Acknowledgements

Chyril Isabel Newitt (nee Henricksen, 29-9-1929 to 10-10-2013), my pioneering mother for her total commitment in giving and sustaining life to the best of her ability

Bernard Stanley Newitt (15-8-1910 to 10-6-1984), my Australian pioneering farmer father for his endurance, persistence, assertiveness and courage improving a large virgin area of land at Waterloo, Monduran Road, within this great country of ours; developing and maintaining a dairy, pig and beef farm (with buildings built from the property's own timber); who commenced and maintained the Yandaran Primary School bus and route from 1957 to 1973; and also begun and drove the Yandaran and District bus run to Kepnock and Bundaberg High Schools from 1964 to 1973; and did the best he knew how at providing what was believed during those years, nutritious food and beverages

My sister, Marie Rose Black (16-4-1951 to 20-7-1998), beloved mother of Kim and Ashley, who gave so much to the youth in Australia and in so doing Marie received the Australian Day Citizen of the Year 1997 Award at Clermont. With her passions towards community spirit, Marie became involved in the Cub Scout Venturer Unit and the Army Cadet Unit where she held the rank of Lieutenant. Her sudden departure from this life at age 47 provided me with much inspiration to place this learned nutritional knowledge, which was created for natural health students, into book form and share with you

The many, many farmers who grow the nutritious foods we all love to be nourished by

My daughters, Sharon and Tina whose spontaneous love is always enjoyed

continued ...

Peter J. E. Hegarty, for editorial assistance and guidance

Stephen R. Hegarty, my husband, for providing me with overwhelming support, encouraging me to follow my dreams

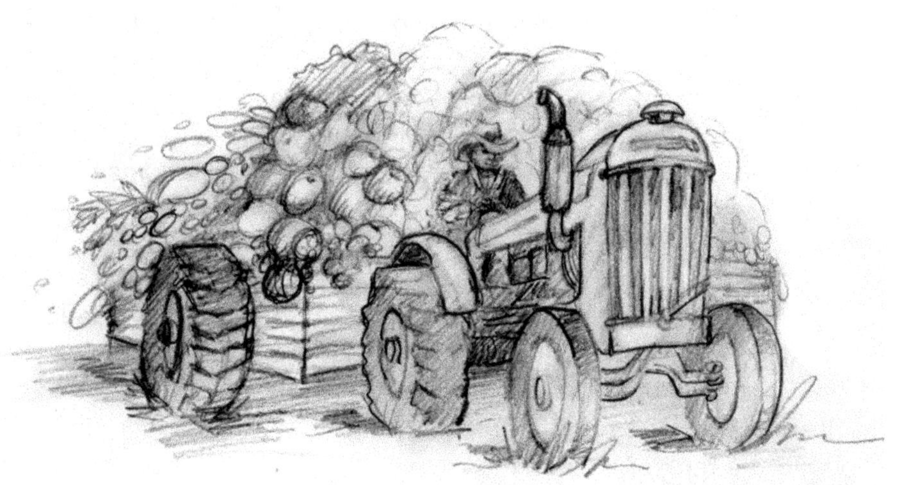

Table of Contents

Foreword

Nutrition is an art as well as a science and Nancy has developed a healthy eating plan for people who differ in their food preferences, beliefs and culture. Food has become our medicine and a majority of people are wanting to educate themselves to eating a healthier diet.

Nancy has excellent qualifications for writing about the nutritional requirements we need for optimum health. Her book, Simple Foods to Heal Your Body, is down to earth, concise and practical, forming a useful reference for the everyday person looking to improve their health and well-being through the food they eat.

Caroline Fisher, Owner/Operator

The Health and Wellness Centre

"Health Healing and Harmony"

Innisfail, Queensland, Australia

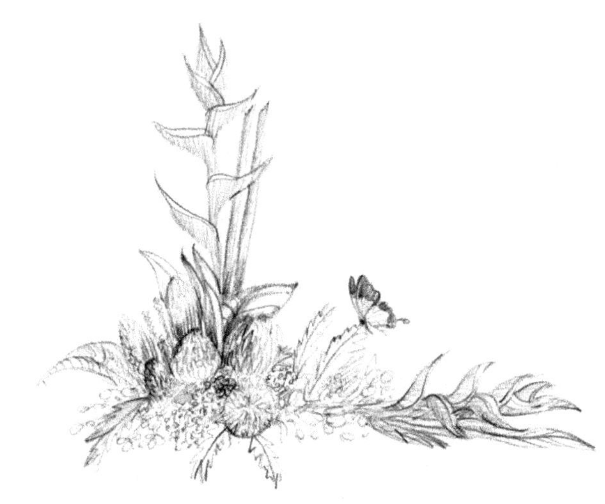

PART 1

INTRODUCTION
THE HEALTHY FACTS OF LIFE
APPROXIMATE DAILY BODY REQUIREMENTS

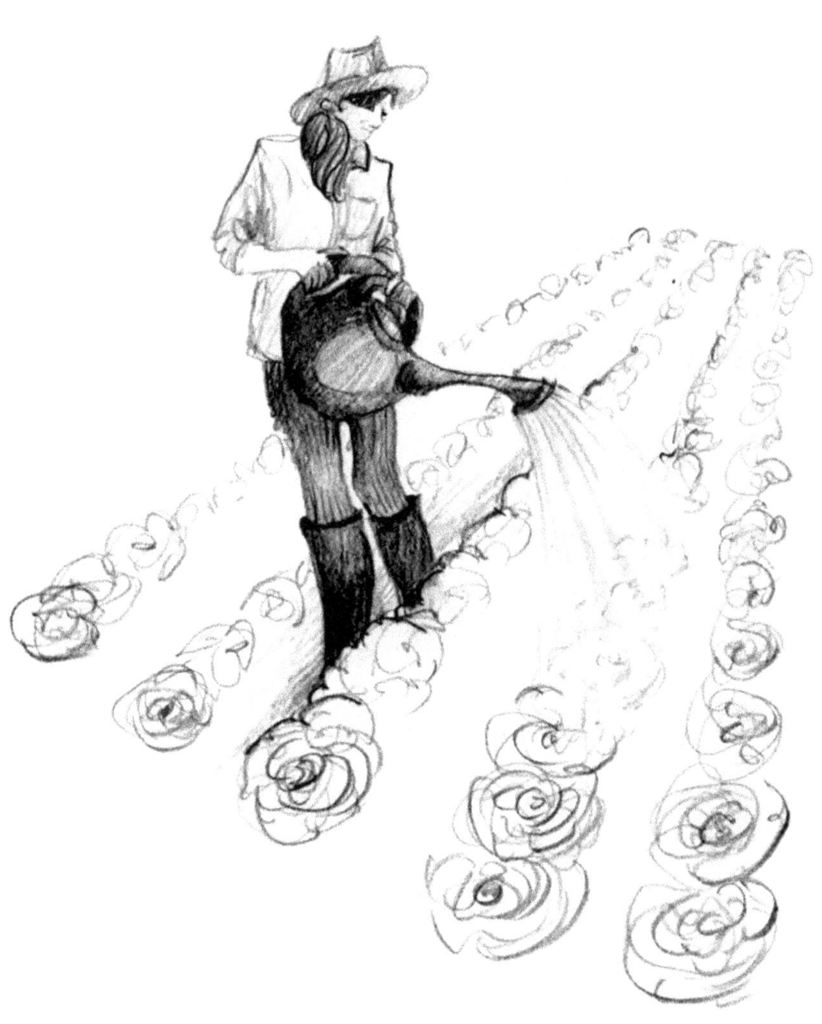

Introduction

What contributes immensely to our moods and general health are the foods we eat, beverages we drink and the buildings we live in. For an agreeable lifestyle, what delightfully goes in can indeed make a favourable impression and besides orally, this includes visually, aromatically, noises within earshot and physical sensations. *Simple Foods to Heal Your Body* shows you the way orally and has the potential to assist with vision, hearing and feelings.

If you hunger for healing an ailment please refer to Part 2, *Ailments from A to Z, Nutrients and Healing Foods* when shopping for delicious, restorative food.

Mouthwatering selections of edibles with high levels of vitamins and/or minerals are located under each ailment.

Choose at least one from each nutrient listed. Remember to select only one ailment and entertain healing it.

Give your body what it needs for healing and not necessarily what your body craves, for example poor eating habits that may have developed from what specific advertisements wanted you to believe or some of your ancestors' 'comfort food' that didn't work for them.

It may take one day or a few, possibly a week or even more before you feel any change and maybe months before you see any differences, however, the sooner you start, the quicker your body can activate the fast-track healing process. Persist and you will succeed in making the best your body can become. Remember that persistence does, in the course of time, lead to success, whether that be this lifetime or the next.

Ensure to start on only one major ailment at a time until that condition has begun to clear. If there are any others, you may find these will simply disappear.

When an ailment has advanced beyond your control, please, for your body's sake, seek professional naturopathic guidance.

A guaranteed process that assists on our pathway to a more healthy life is self-love. Access is readily available because we desire more time and energy for our life's purpose while enjoying being on this planet.

Loving everything we consume, having fun along our life's journey, delighting in a little play each day and loving what we do all position our bodies on the speedy track for upgraded health.

Before discovering which food to eat for this or that, I have introduced a snippet of metaphysics in *The Healthy Facts Of Life* to prepare you for what is approaching next. Understanding how our bodies react to certain stimuli provides a greater awareness, and therefore with this knowledge healing can be accomplished to a large extent with less difficulty. Healing takes effort. From your determined attempts rewards begin to appear. If it becomes too overwhelming for you, simply move onto Approximate Daily Adult Body Requirements or Ailments, Nutrients and Healing Foods. Love your body for all that it is now and please take pleasure from all that you create.

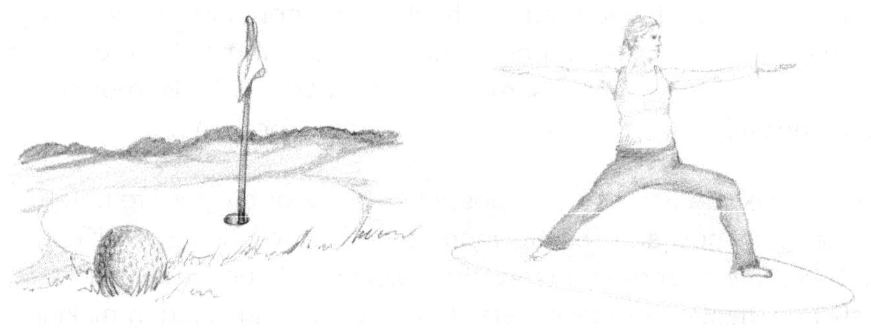

Aging is optional

The Healthy Facts Of Life

Breathing, eating, exercise and rest are life. What we breathe, eat and do with our bodies is mostly in our hands and at our feet. If you can read this, then you also have control over your bodily intake. If you have a body that is in pain, then its intelligence is saying, "STOP! What you are doing is hurting me! Please change the way you treat me."

The best place to start is by saying and repeating this affirmation over and over until it begins to feel true for you and ***feel*** what your body has to say about it. "I am healthy." It does not matter if this is not true right now. If there is any negative thought coming to mind then you know you need to overcome that to produce the outcome, "I am healthy." This is your ***new goal***, "I am healthy," your new direction. By continuing whining to yourself or anyone who cannot help your problem to change you will never be healed. Your body cells need to know exactly what they have to do for you.

As your body makes changes to new ways of thinking, more than likely you may feel like rejecting these new ideas and beliefs because you have never thought this way before.

You are now in control of your body and you know that it is only change. You are willing to change old ideas and beliefs that have not previously worked for you. You own your body, no-one else, and it is divinely gifted to you to protect and feed with nourishing foods and beverages. Sit ever so quietly and think about these questions. Listen to what your own body cells are telling you.

- How does your food taste in its natural state?
- Are there any that come to mind that you eat but dislike?
- Do you enjoy its individual flavor?
- Does any of your food need to be disguised just to make it palatable?

- Could you eat this food with no additives?
- If not, why not?
- If not, why do you need to eat or drink it?

Balancing your body does not require a degree however it does take awareness and persistence. I repeat, the best place to start is by saying this affirmation over and over, with lots of emphasis,

"I AM HEALTHY"

Continue repeating this affirmation until you begin to ***feel*** it is true. Your body *knows* what is right for it and in the event that you feed it more than it requires of certain ingredients, you *will* feel it and you will *know* it!

Print "I AM HEALTHY" neatly onto a piece of paper and place this onto your bathroom mirror where, looking into your eyes every time you see it, you can say "I am healthy" to re-program your body cells. If you feel no reaction to this statement than you must already have a healthy body and therefore do not need to do this exercise.

Many nutrition cookery books have been written by people who at one time were very ill and worked out a system that healed their illness. This does not work for everyone; e.g. people who follow the Paleo diet eat lots of grass fed meats, poultry, fish, seafood, non-starchy vegetables and fruits, nuts and seeds; raw food people eat all their food raw, seldom eat grains and are careful not to eat vegetables and fruits at the same meal and never eat salt, and there are the macrobiotic people who cook nearly everything, combine food differently and use lots of salt. You will find many books on the topic of nutrition.

A high content of nutrients is removed from whole grains during the process into white flour, therefore some whole grains are nutritiously beneficial. As you will see there are considerably large quantities of nutrients, especially vitamin E in whole meal.

If you eat refined flours, your body will take a few weeks to adjust to whole grains. Digestion is made easier by grinding the grains to flour prior to cooking. If it is your skin that requires change, your skin will love you for this change (for example: less pimples, less dryness, less cracks, less sores and boils), improved muscle tone with a daily exercise regime, improved teeth and bones when combined with magnesium, shinier hair and so on it goes to boundless energy. These are clearly a few of the new changes you may experience.

If you notice a pimple or rash, discover or re-discover an enjoyable hobby, eliminate the sweet foods. Enjoy a rest daily and drink more naturally oxygenated and finely filtered rain water until it disappears.

As your body adapts to its healthier way of eating, you will create your own recipes and adapt these for your personal requirements and enjoyment. You will discover that this is easy and fun to do. You may like to begin by exchanging white flours for whole-meal flours, using ½ and ½, then go on to replacing white flour entirely for whole-meal flour. For your heart's sake you may like to try flaxseed, soybean, corn, coconut or safflower oils in raw salads. Two of the most impressive advancements are the breathing capacity and the control over your body's functions. Your entire body will love you for this new way of dining.

If your body has been unaccustomed to eating unrefined foods, then this change will take some time for your body to adjust to a new way of consuming nourishment. The transition is well worth the persistence and the long-term benefits. Your intestines will feel different because you will be awakening or re-building the muscles. Gas may form. The stomach may feel bloated.

Have no fear. It is only the change process occurring. Wholesome food is much more beneficial to your body and you need less. As you gently rub your abdomen, try the following new positive affirmation and, if necessary, repeat many times until it settles:

"I RELAX, LETTING LIFE FLOW EASILY THROUGH ME"

Your skin may also feel different; dry, flaky, pimply or cracked, or maybe oily. This is quite normal as the seborrhea regulation process adjusts. A good affirmation to use often is:

"I ACCEPT MYSELF WHERE I AM RIGHT NOW KNOWING I AM SAFE"

Your body may start to act differently. Do not be alarmed by some of the unusual things you may do. This is only from the change process occurring. Your body has been told to do something completely opposite to what it has known in the past. Your brain wants to stay in the past because it feels safer there with what it already knows then to move forward not knowing if it will succeed. It is known as the fear of failure. You can succeed and you will thrive and prosper. Each time a negative thought comes into your head, counteract it and reassure your body,

"I AM BALANCED AND DOING THE BEST I CAN FOR MY BODY."

How is your body reacting? Is it beginning to resist change?

- Is your body getting irritated in any way?
- Is your body itching (feeling threatened)?
- Is your body developing a headache (doesn't like this new pressure)?
- Are your eyes feeling different (don't want to look at this)?
- What do your ears feel like – ringing noise or aches (don't want to hear this)?

How tight is your:

- Jaw (any anger there or feelings of indecision)?
- Neck (feeling inflexible or stubborn about any change)?
- Back (fear of no support either emotionally or financially)?
- Stomach (fear of the new)?

How tight are your:

- Fingers or toes (concerned with the little details)?
- Shoulders (carrying burdens)?

- ◑ Genitals (concerned about not being good enough)?
- ◑ Knees (unable to bend and won't give in to change)?
- ◑ Ankles (fear of changing directions)?

These are a few of the ways your body 'talks' to you when it is not happy with what is going on around it and within it. Any of these reactions is good. This is an awareness step in your healing process.

By being aware you can now begin your healing or changing old negative patterns. When you mention a condition, complain about it or see it in other people, you also begin to relate to it.

Now that you know what your body loves, you can help it through this process and I will guide you. Deep within your subconscious mind you know automatically what is best for your body.

Here are a few questions to ponder over.

- ▼ How were you fed as a child?
- ▼ How did your body look then?
- ▼ How does it look now?
- ▼ Is your diet different now to when you were growing into an adult?
- ▼ How did your parents look, and your grandparents, if you saw them?
- ▼ If they are still living, how do they look now?
- ▼ How would you like to look when you are elderly?

Parents have taught us many ways that have helped us to where we are today. They are also open to learning new ways of living too. No matter how you are today, your ancestors did the very best they could using the knowledge, understanding and awareness they had. Some nutritional knowledge was only becoming available to the public from around the 1960s. Every day knowledge continues to be uncovered and shared for our life's enjoyment.

Firstly, you need to know a little about what your body's daily requirements are. Following is a guide for you and is not always true for everyone. Your body may already be seriously low in any one nutrient or more. If in doubt then please consult your nearest naturopath or nutritionist. Allow your body to display to you what it needs. Listen to its urges and demands. Your subconscious mind knows what is good for your body so ***feel*** your body's answers. Every cell has its own Divine intelligence. You ***will*** recognize the signs and the correct answers. Perform these accordingly for your magnificent body and it will happily respond.

If you have been diagnosed with an allergy to a particular item, simply delete it or substitute with another of similar characteristics (e.g. if you have an allergy to dairy milk – try coconut, soy, rice or almond milk, if you must have some form of milk). If you are unsure, a professional kinesiologist can perform non-invasive muscle testing.

For bodily moisturising, drink up to two litres of finely filtered or boiled water each day. The amount will depend upon your activities and climate, and ease up on sweet foods if your lips, eyes or skin feel/s dry or sticky, especially when you awaken in the mornings.

If your skin is itching excessively, eat lots of green leafy vegetables for that day.

If you eat meat and your body feels excessively tired, cease eating meat for that day and cut back on the daily quantity to a portion size of 125 grams or less.

If your body feels bloated, eliminate grains for that day, including breads and especially cakes and biscuits.

If your gums have receded and food particles become trapped between your teeth use dental floss after each meal. It is best to remove leftover food rather than leave it there to rot, produce bad breath and harmful bacteria that can end up going through your entire digestive system creating an ill feeling in the abdomen. Gently brush your teeth twice daily.

Discover the taste of real food by trying some of the many delicious nutrient-rich recipes available. You will discover lots in nutrition books. Enjoy their delights and share these around with your friends.

The speed of any recovery will entirely depend upon the amount of effort you are prepared to put into this life changing event for your loved ones and your country.

Now let's move on with nutrient requirements. Protein, next to water, is the most plentiful substance in the body. Most meats and dairy products are complete-protein foods, whilst most vegetables and fruits are incomplete-protein foods. Protein is necessary for growth and development and acts in the formation of hormones, enzymes and antibodies. Protein also maintains acid-alkali balance and is a source of heat and energy.

Carbohydrates provide energy for body functions and muscular exertions, assisting in digestion and assimilation of foods.

Fat provides energy and acts as a carrier for fat-soluble vitamins A, D, E, and K, supplying essential fatty acids needed for growth, health, and smooth skin.

There is so much information out there about cholesterol. Here's some more that you may find useful. It is a fat-related substance necessary for good health, being a normal component of most body tissues, especially those of the brain and nervous system, liver and blood; needed to form sex and adrenal hormones, vitamin D, and bile which is needed for the digestion of fats. Eat fats sparingly. Enjoying raw salad vegetables or a raw fruit portion with a small amount of fat can make the digestion process more enjoyable.

For fitness enhancement add a daily serving of fresh sprouts. Your body becomes more energetic and your brain thinks more clearly. Everything begins to function better. Some sprouts such as mung beans are so easy to grow in the kitchen. There are good indoor gardening books that can assist in this area.

You may also like to travel in order to learn about food that is consumed in other countries. See what culinary delights each country's residents enjoy and take note of their fitness. Have fun and enjoy learning what each nutrient (or lack of) does and can do for your body.

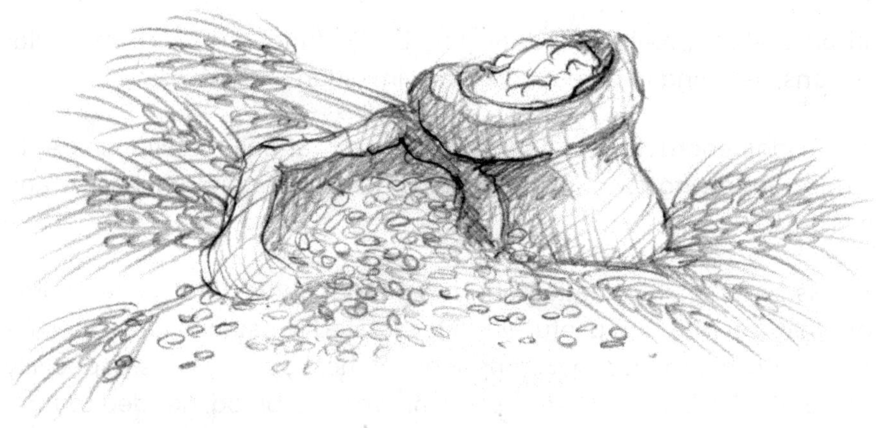

Approximate Daily Adult Body Requirements

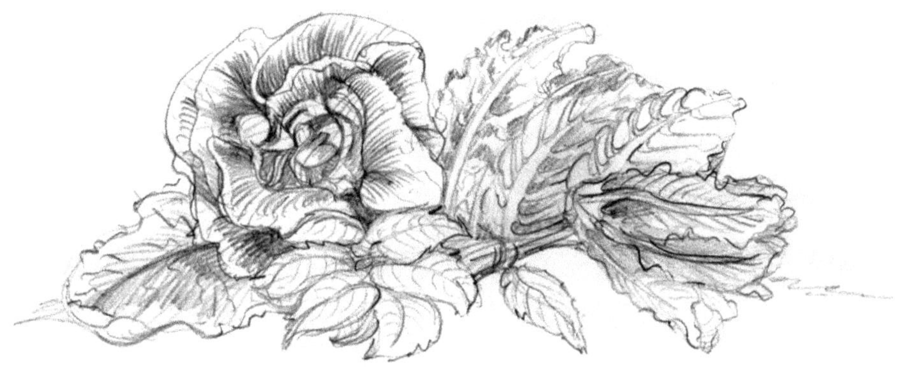

Research indicates the daily body requirements for adults, and children from four years of age are as follows: (Obtain medical advice for babies, infants, pregnant or lactating women)

BIOFLAVONOIDS

Vitamin P - no recommended daily allowance - Help increase strength of capillaries - Protective agent against harmful effects of x-rays; lowers tendency to bleed, hemorrhage or bruise easily

Best Sources: buckwheat, grapes, plums, blackcurrants, apricots, cherries, blackberries, lemons, rose hips

CALCIUM

800 mg - Treats rheumatism, output of estrogen, premenstrual tension, menstrual cramps, "growing pains;" essential for healthy blood; eases insomnia; helps regulate heartbeat

Best Sources: milk, milk products, green leafy vegetables, shellfish, molasses

CHLORINE

Chloride - no recommended daily allowance - Helps regulate correct acid and alkaline balance in the blood; stimulates hydrochloric acid needed in the stomach for digestion of protein, and rough, fibrous foods; stimulates the liver to function as a filter and helps clean toxic wastes out of the body. Chlorine in drinking water destroys vitamin E and also destroys many of the intestinal flora that help in food digestion

Best Sources: sea salt, kelp, rye flour, dulse, ripe olives, sea greens, and most foods

CHROMIUM

.05 mg to .2 mg - Stimulates activity of enzymes involved in the metabolism of glucose for energy and the synthesis of fatty acids and cholesterol; helps regulate sugar in the blood

Best Sources: brewer's yeast, whole grains, whole wheat bread, liver, beef, beets, beet sugar molasses, grapes, mushrooms

COPPER

2 mg - With iron forms hemoglobin; aids in the conversion of amino acid tyrosine into a dark pigment that colours hair and skin; and helps the body to oxidize vitamin C, working with C in the formation of elastin, the chief component of elastic muscle fibres; is necessary for proper bone formation and maintenance

Best Sources: seafood, organ meats, almonds, legumes, green leafy vegetables, molasses, raisins, whole grains

FOLIC ACID

Folacin - .4 mg - Deficiency may lead to forgetfulness, mental sluggishness, irritability; Oral contraceptives and sulphur drugs may interfere with absorption

Best Sources: dark green leafy vegetables, organ meats, root vegetables, whole grains, oysters, salmon, milk

BIOTIN

.3 mg - Improves dermatitis; treats depression and muscle pain

Best Sources: egg yolks, liver, unpolished rice, whole grains, sardines, legumes

CHOLINE

No recommended daily allowance however that average daily diet yields between 500 and 900mg - Prevents fats from accumulating in the kidney, facilitating movement of fats into the cells; helps regulate and improve liver and gallbladder functioning and aids in prevention of gallstones; utilizes fats and cholesterol in the body

Best Sources: egg yolk, liver, brewer's yeast, wheat germ

FLUORINE

Fluorides 1.5 to 4 mg - Increases the deposition of calcium, thereby strengthening bones; helps reduce formation of acid in the mouth caused by carbohydrates. High levels of fluorides can depress growth, cause calcification of ligaments and tendons, and mottle teeth

Best Sources: tea, seafood, cheese, meat

INOSITOL

No recommended daily allowance however that average daily diet yields about 1 gm - Helps lower cholesterol levels in blood; relieves mild hypertension; eliminates need for sedatives

Best Sources: unprocessed whole grains, citrus fruits, brewer's yeast, molasses, liver

IRON

18 mg - Iron-deficiency anaemia needs a diet high in iron rich foods along with vitamin C to speed up restoration of hemoglobin levels to normal.

Best Sources: organ meats, meats, eggs, fish, poultry, molasses, cherry juice, green leafy vegetables, dried fruits, parsley

IODINE

Iodide - 150 mcg - Deficiency may result in cretinism, hardening of the arteries; thyroid enlargement and hypothyroidism

Best Sources: seafood, kelp

MAGNESIUM

400 mg - Helps form the kind of hard tooth enamel that resists decay – only a soft enamel will form without magnesium; helps to protect the accumulation of calcium deposits in the urinary tract; makes calcium and phosphorus soluble in urine and prevents them from turning into hard stones; helps control delirium tremens; helps keep arteries healthy; treats painful uterine contractions; acts as antacid

Best Sources: seafood, whole grains, dark green vegetables, molasses, oil-rich seeds and nuts, especially almonds, raw unmilled wheat germ, figs, corn, apples, soybeans, milk

MANGANESE

2.5 to 5 mg - Helps nourish brain and nerves; maintain sex-hormone production; essential for the formation of thyroxin, a constituent of the thyroid gland; Deficiency may effect glucose tolerance resulting in the inability to remove excess sugar from the blood by oxidation causing diabetes; is effective in increasing copper excretion from schizophrenics

Best Sources: whole grains, green leafy vegetables, legumes, nuts, pineapples, egg yolks, seeds

MOLYBDENUM

.15 mg to .5 mg - Deficiency may result in male impotence

Best Sources: meats, legumes, whole grains, dark-green leafy vegetables

PANGAMIC ACID

B15 - no recommended daily allowance - Stimulates glandular and nervous system; promotes protein metabolism; regulates fat and sugar metabolism

Best Sources: apricot kernels, whole brown rice, whole grain cereals, sesame seeds, pumpkin seeds, in crystalline from rice bran, rice polish, and brewer's yeast

PANTOTHENIC ACID

B5 - 10 mg - Helps build antibodies for fighting infection; greatest defense against stress and fatigue; stimulates adrenal glands and increases production of cortisone and other adrenal hormones important for healthy nerves and skin; relieves intestinal gas and abdominal distension; destroyed by acid such as vinegar, or alkali such as baking soda

Best Sources: organ meats, egg yolks, legumes, whole grains, wheat germ, salmon

PARA-AMINOBENZOIC ACID

PABA - no recommended daily allowance - Helps restore colour to hair; alleviates the pain of sunburn; treats schizophrenia, and vitiligo (pigmentation)

Best Sources: liver, yeast, wheat germ, and molasses

PHOSPHORUS

800 mg - Speeds up the healing process in bone fractures and also reduces the loss of calcium in such; Deficiency in the calcium-phosphorus balance may result in arthritis, rickets, pyorrhea, and tooth decay

Best Sources: fish, meat, poultry, eggs, nuts, seeds, whole grains

POTASSIUM

1875mg to 5625 mg - Assists in conversion of glucose into glycogen; stimulates kidneys to eliminate poisonous body wastes; treats high blood pressure directly caused by excessive salt intake; essential for the transmission of nerve impulses to the brain

Best Sources: lean meats, whole grains, vegetables, especially green leafy vegetables, potatoes, oranges, bananas, dried fruits, legumes, sunflower seeds, mint leaves

SELENIUM

0.5 to .2 mg - Deficiency results in infertility

Best Sources: tuna, herring, brewer's yeast, wheat germ and bran, whole grains, sesame seeds, organ and muscle meats, dairy products, shellfish

SULPHUR

Treats arthritis, and skin disorders - There is no recommended daily requirement. If sufficient protein is consumed there is also enough sulphur.

Best Sources: eggs, meat, fish, cheese, milk

UNSATURATED FATTY ACIDS

No recommended daily allowance however intake is best to not exceed 10% of total calories - Important for respiration of vital organs; helps maintain resilience and lubrication; Deficiency symptoms are brittle and lusterless hair, brittle nails and dandruff

Best Sources: vegetable oils, sunflower seeds

VANADIUM

100 mcg to 300 mcg - Deficiency may result in decreased reproduction rates and increased mortality in the young

Best Sources: whole grains, seafood, liver, meats

VITAMIN A

4000 I.U. - Protects the epithelial tissues like the skin, stomach, and lungs from becoming cancerous; helps fight infections by protecting the mucous membranes against invading bacteria; Deficiency leads to rapid loss of vitamin C.

Best Sources: Liver, eggs, orange and yellow vegetables and fruits, dark green leafy vegetables, whole milk, milk products

VITAMIN B1

Thiamine - 1.5 mg - Improves muscle tone in the stomach and intestines thereby relieving constipation; improves individual learning capacity; improves muscle tone in the heart; destroyed by an enzyme present in raw oysters, raw fish and raw clams

Best Sources: whole grains, molasses, brown rice, organ meats, meats, fish, poultry, egg yolks, legumes, nuts

VITAMIN B2

Riboflavin - 1.7 mg – Improves cell respiration, working with enzymes in the utilization of cell oxygen; maintains good vision, skin, nails, and hair

Best Sources: whole grains, molasses, organ meats, egg yolks, legumes, nuts

VITAMIN B3

Niacin - 20 mg - Stimulates production of hydrochloric acid to aid impaired digestion; widens blood vessels; increases joint mobility

Best Sources: lean meats, poultry, fish, peanuts, milk, milk products, rice bran

VITAMIN B6

Pyridoxine - 2 mg - Treats muscular weakness, burning feet, acne; prevents water build-up in tissues; controls nausea and vomiting during pregnancy; reduces pain and size of reddened knots on the sides of finger joints during menopause; treats photosensitivity to sunlight

Best Sources: meats, whole grains, organ meats, molasses, wheat germ, legumes, green leafy vegetables

VITAMIN B12

6 mcg - Reduces effects of bruising and black eyes; treats hangovers; Deficiency may cause mental deterioration and paralysis.

Best Sources: organ meats, muscle meats, fish, pork, milk products

VITAMIN C

60 mg - Promotes fine bone and tooth formation; speeds up the healing of wounds - bleeding may continue or restart if insufficient C is not available for wound healing. Excess bicarbonate of soda in the system can destroy vitamin C.

Best Sources: raw papaya or pawpaw, acerola cherries, capsicum, strawberries, tangerine juice, pineapple, orange juice, rose hips, alfalfa sprouts, broccoli, tomato, mango, cantaloupe, grapefruit juice, kiwi fruit and all raw vegetables, fruits and edible herbs

VITAMIN D

400 I.U. - Aids the absorption of calcium from the intestinal tract, and the breakdown and assimilation of phosphorus that is required for bone formation; helps prevent tooth decay; Vitamins D with A are beneficial in reducing colds and with vitamin C act as a preventative measure.

Best Sources: Salmon, sardines, herring, egg yolks, organ meats, sunlight (approximately 10 minutes daily where possible, preferably early morning, before 8.00am (this of course will depend on where you live, and avoid sunburn).

VITAMIN E

Tocopherol - 30 I.U. - Works with vitamin C to keep blood vessels flexible, healthy; increases male and female fertility. Estrogen is a vitamin E antagonist. Chlorine in drinking water, ferric chloride, rancid oil or fat, and inorganic iron compounds destroy vitamin E in the body. Deficiency is the rupture of red blood cells, broken capillaries.

Best Sources: cold-pressed oils of wheat germ, soybean and corn, wheat germ, molasses, sweet potato, leafy vegetables

VITAMIN K

No recommended daily allowance however an average daily intake is estimated between 300 and 500 mcg - Reduces blood flow and clots during prolonged menstruation; reduces blood loss; Destroyed by rancid fats, radiation, aspirin, industrial air pollution

Best Sources: kelp, alfalfa, green plants, leafy green vegetables, cow's milk, yogurt, egg yolks, molasses, safflower oil, fish-liver oils

ZINC

15 mg - Eliminates cholesterol deposits; helps heal wounds; helps prevent and treat infertility; reduces body odour

Best Sources: oysters (cooked), pumpkin seeds, sunflower seeds, seafood, organ meats, mushrooms, soybeans, herring, eggs, wheat germ, meats

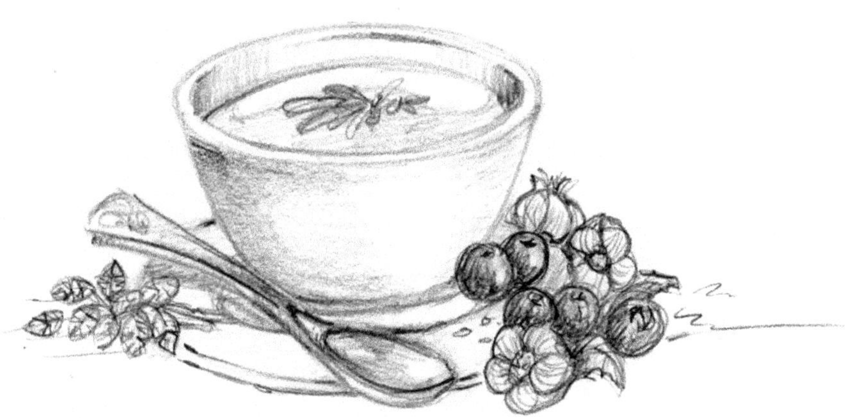

PART 2

AILMENTS FROM A TO Z, NUTRIENTS AND HEALING FOODS

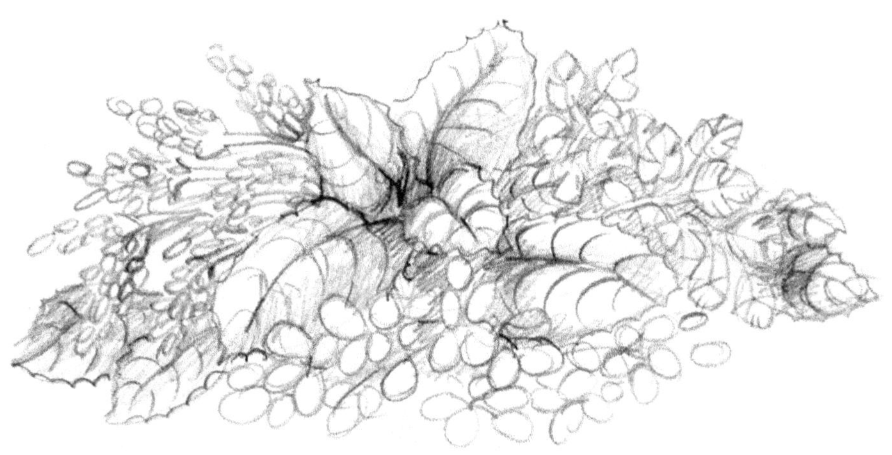

Ailments from A to Z, Nutrients and Healing Foods

Choose only one ailment at a time and for at least one month commence eating your body's natural healing foods. If the ailment has only one nutrient listed, add green leafy vegetables, raw sprouts and filtered rainwater to your diet and see a health physician for more advice, especially with regards to any possible food allergies.

If you have more than one ailment to commence healing, you may even discover what you eat for one may also be healing any other ailments. Enjoy eating simple foods that heal your body.

ABSCESS

A (unprocessed orange fruits and vegetables), B group (whole grains i.e. whole or ground wheat, whole or ground brown rice), C (raw fruits and vegetables), E (cold-pressed oils, eggs, wheat germ), filtered, detoxified rainwater

ACCIDENTS, SHOCK, SURGERY

B group (whole or ground wheat, whole or ground brown rice), C (raw fruits and vegetables), E (cold-pressed oils, eggs, wheat germ), Protein (lean meat, fish, poultry, soybeans, eggs, milk, whole grains, skim yogurt), B2 (whole grains, egg yolk, legumes, nuts), B6 (lean meats, whole grains, wheat germ, legumes, green leafy vegetables), Folic Acid (dark green leafy vegetables, root vegetables, whole grains, oysters, salmon, milk), Pantothenic Acid (including egg yolk, legumes, whole grains, wheat germ, salmon), D (salmon, sardines, herrings), Calcium (skim milk, green leafy vegetables, shellfish), Copper (seafood, nuts, legumes, raisins), Magnesium (seafood, whole grains, dark green vegetables, nuts), Zinc (pumpkin seeds, sunflower seeds, seafood, mushrooms, soybeans, oysters, herring, eggs, wheat germ, lean meat)

ACNE

A (unprocessed orange vegetables and fruits), B Group (whole grains i.e. whole or ground wheat, whole or ground brown rice), C (raw fruits and vegetables), E (cold-pressed vegetable oils, eggs, wheat germ), Zinc (pumpkin seeds, sunflower seeds, seafood, mushrooms, soybeans, oysters, herring, egg, wheat germ, lean meats), B2 (including wild rice, almonds, venison), B6 (brown rice, pinto beans, trout, sunflower seeds), Niacin (peanuts, rice bran, trout, salmon, rabbit, pheasant, quail), Pantothenic Acid (peanuts, plain skim yogurt, sunflower seeds, mushrooms, pinto beans, corn, abalone, lobster, salmon, trout, dark chicken meat, pheasant), C (raw fruits and vegetables), E (cold-pressed vegetable oils, eggs, wheat germ), Zinc (pumpkin seeds, sunflower seeds, seafood, mushrooms, soybeans, oysters, herring, egg, wheat germ, lean meats), D (salmon, sardines, herrings), Unsaturated fatty acids (vegetable oils, sunflower seeds), Calcium (skim milk, green leafy vegetables, shellfish), Potassium (lean meats, whole grains, vegetables, legumes, dried fruits, sunflower seeds), Sulphur (fish, red peppers, garlic, onions, eggs, lean meats, cabbage, brussel sprouts, horseradish)

ACQUIRED IMMUNODEFICIENCY SYNDROME

A (unprocessed orange vegetables and fruits), E (cold-pressed vegetable oils, eggs, wheat germ), C (raw fruits and vegetables), B12 (fish, pork, eggs, milk), B6 (brown rice, pinto beans, trout, sunflower seeds), Folic Acid (dark green vegetables, root vegetables, whole grains, oysters, salmon, milk)

ADRENAL EXHAUSTION

B group (whole or ground wheat, whole or ground brown rice), B2 (wild rice, almonds, venison), B12 (fish, pork, eggs, milk), Folic Acid (dark green vegetables, root vegetables, whole grains, oysters, salmon, milk), Pantothenic Acid (egg yolk, legumes, whole grains, wheat germ, salmon), C (raw fruits and vegetables), E (cold-pressed vegetable oils, eggs, wheat germ), Potassium (lean meats, whole grains, vegetables, legumes, dried fruits, sunflower seeds), Sodium (seafood, sea salt, celery, milk products, kelp), Unsaturated fatty acids (vegetable oils, sunflower seeds)

ALCOHOLISM

A (unprocessed orange vegetables and fruits), B group (whole or ground wheat, whole or ground brown rice), B1 (whole grains, lean meats, fish, poultry, egg yolks), B2 (whole grains, egg yolks, legumes, nuts), B6 (lean meats, whole grains, wheat germ, legumes, green leafy vegetables), B12 (fish, pork, eggs, low salt cheese, milk), Choline (egg yolks, unpolished rice, whole grains, sardines, legumes), Folic Acid (dark green vegetables, root vegetables, whole grains, oysters, salmon, milk), Niacin (peanuts, rice bran, trout, salmon, rabbit, pheasant, quail), Pangamic Acid (brown rice, sunflower seeds, pumpkin seeds, sesame seeds), Pantothenic Acid (egg yolks, legumes, whole grains, wheat germ, salmon), C (raw fruits and vegetables), D (salmon, sardines, herrings, egg yolks, organ meats), E (cold-pressed vegetable oils, eggs, wheat germ), K (green leafy vegetables, egg yolks, safflower oil, cauliflower, soybeans), Chromium (grapes, raisins, corn oil, clams, whole grains), Iron (lean meats, eggs, fish, poultry, cherry juice, green leafy vegetables), Magnesium (seafood, whole grains, dark green vegetables, nuts), Manganese (whole grains, green leafy vegetables, legumes, nuts, pineapple, egg yolk), Zinc (pumpkin seeds, sunflower seeds, seafood, mushrooms, soybeans, oysters, herring, egg, wheat germ, lean meats), Unsaturated fatty acids (vegetable oils, sunflower seeds)

ALLERGIES

A (unprocessed orange vegetables and fruits), B group (whole grains i.e. whole or ground wheat, whole or ground brown rice), B6 (lean meats, whole grains, wheat germ, legumes, green leafy vegetables), B12 (fish, pork, eggs, low salt cheese, milk), Niacin (peanuts, rice bran, trout, salmon, rabbit, pheasant, quail), Pantothenic Acid (egg yolks, legumes, whole grains, wheat germ, salmon), C (raw fruits and vegetables), D (salmon, sardines, herrings, egg yolks, organ meats), E (cold-pressed vegetable oils, eggs, wheat germ), Unsaturated fatty acids (vegetable oils, sunflower seeds), Calcium (skim milk, green leafy vegetables, shellfish), Magnesium (seafood, whole grains, dark green vegetables, nuts), Manganese (whole grains, green leafy vegetables, legumes, nuts, pineapple, egg yolk)

ANAEMIA

B group (whole grains i.e. whole or ground wheat, whole or ground brown rice), B1 (whole grains, lean meats, fish, poultry, egg yolks), B6 (lean meats, whole grains, wheat germ, legumes, green leafy vegetables), B12 (fish, pork, eggs, low salt cheese, milk), Folic Acid (dark-green vegetables, root vegetables, whole grains, oysters, salmon, milk), PABA (wheat germ, yeast, molasses, liver), Pantothenic Acid (egg yolks, legumes, whole grains, wheat germ, salmon), C (raw fruits and vegetables), E (cold-pressed vegetable oils, eggs, wheat germ), Calcium (skim milk, green leafy vegetables, shellfish), Cobalt (oysters, clams, poultry, milk, green leafy vegetables, fruits), Copper (seafood, nuts, legumes, raisins), Iron (meat, eggs, fish, poultry, cherry juice, green leafy vegetables, dried fruits), Magnesium (seafood, whole grains, dark green vegetables, nuts), Protein (meat, fish, poultry, soybeans, eggs, milk, whole grains)

ANAEMIA, COPPER DEFICIENCY

Copper (seafood, nuts, legumes, raisins)

ANAEMIA, FOLIC ACID DEFICIENCY

Folic Acid (dark green vegetables, root vegetables, whole grains, oysters, salmon, milk); Present with Tropical Sprue, some pregnant women and infants born to deficient mothers, and alcoholics

ANAEMIA, MEGALOBLASTIC

B group (whole grains i.e. whole or ground wheat, whole or ground brown rice), Folic Acid (dark green vegetables, root vegetables, whole grains, oysters, salmon, milk)

Please note: Underlying abnormality actually shows as a B12 and Folic Acid deficiency

ANAEMIA OF PROTEIN-ENERGY MALNUTRITION

Protein (meat, fish, poultry, soybeans, eggs, milk, whole grains), Iron (lean meats, eggs, fish, poultry, cherry juice, green leafy vegetables), Folic Acid (dark green vegetables, root vegetables, whole grains, oysters, salmon, milk)

ANAEMIA, VITAMIN E-RESPONSIVE

E (wheat germ, eggs, sweet potato, leafy vegetables, cucumber cold-pressed vegetable oils)

ANOREXIA NERVOSA

Suggestions: *Daily Relaxation Meditation* or *Pain Management & Preparation for Healing Meditation* (see Best from the Library)

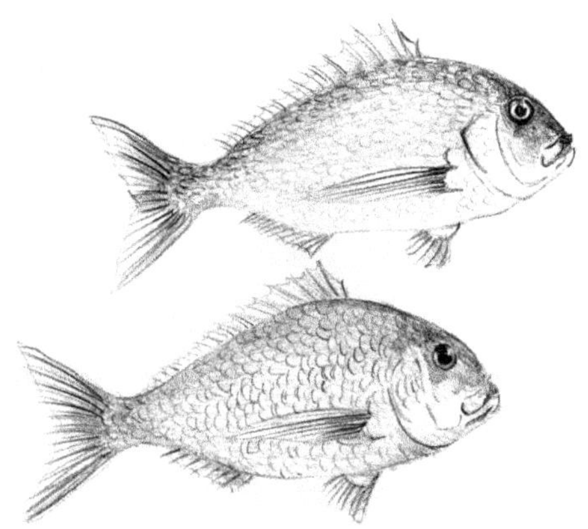

ARTERIOSCLEROSIS & ATHEROSCLEROSIS

A (unprocessed orange vegetables and fruits), B group (whole grains i.e. whole or ground wheat, whole or ground brown rice), B6 (lean meats, whole grains, wheat germ, legumes, green leafy vegetables), B12 (fish, pork, eggs, low salt cheese, milk), Choline (egg yolks, unpolished rice, whole grains, sardines, legumes), Folic Acid (dark green vegetables, root vegetables, whole grains, oysters, salmon, milk), Inositol (whole grains, citrus fruits, meat, milk, nuts, vegetables), Niacin (peanuts, rice bran, trout, salmon, rabbit, pheasant, quail), C (raw fruits and vegetables), E (cold-pressed vegetable oils, eggs, wheat germ), Bioflavonoids (unprocessed citrus fruits, fruits, blackcurrants, buckwheat), Calcium (skim milk, green leafy vegetables, shellfish), Chromium (grapes, raisins, corn oil, clams, whole grains), Cobalt (oysters, clams, poultry, milk, green leafy vegetables, fruits), Iodine (seafood, kelp), Iron (meat, eggs, fish, poultry, cherry juice, green leafy vegetables, dried fruits), Magnesium (seafood, whole grains, dark green vegetables, nuts), Manganese (whole grains, green leafy vegetables, legumes, nuts, pineapple, egg yolk), Pectin (citrus fruits, apples), Phosphorus (fish, lean meat, poultry, eggs, milk, nuts, whole grains), Potassium (lean meats, whole grains, vegetables, dried fruits, legumes, sunflower seeds), Selenium (tuna, herring, wheat germ, wheat bran, whole grains, sunflower seeds), Vanadium (fish), Zinc (pumpkin seeds, sunflower seeds, seafood, mushrooms, soybeans, oysters, herring, eggs, wheat germ, lean meat)

ARTHRITIS

A (unprocessed orange vegetables and fruits), B group (whole grains i.e. whole or ground wheat, whole or ground brown rice), B2 (whole grains, egg yolks, legumes, nuts), B6 (lean meats, whole grains, wheat germ, legumes, green leafy vegetables), B12 (fish, pork, eggs, low salt cheese, milk), Folic Acid (dark green vegetables, root vegetables, whole grains, oysters, salmon, milk), Inositol (whole grains, citrus fruits, meat, milk, nuts, vegetables), Niacin (peanuts, rice bran, trout, salmon, rabbit, pheasant, quail), PABA (wheat germ, yogurt, green leafy vegetables. molasses), Pantothenic Acid (egg yolks, legumes, whole grains, wheat germ, salmon), C (raw fruits and vegetables), D (salmon, sardines, herrings, egg yolks, organ meats), E (cold-pressed vegetable oils, eggs, wheat germ), Unsaturated Fatty Acids (vegetable oils, sunflower seeds), Bioflavonoids (unprocessed citrus fruits, fruits, blackcurrants, buckwheat), Calcium (skim milk, green leafy vegetables, shellfish), Copper (seafood, nuts, legumes, raisins), Iodine (seafood, kelp), Magnesium (seafood, whole grains, dark green vegetables, nuts), Manganese (whole grains, green leafy vegetables, legumes, nuts, pineapple, egg yolk), Phosphorus (fish, lean meat, poultry, eggs, milk, nuts, whole grains), Potassium (lean meats, whole grains, vegetables, dried fruits, legumes, sunflower seeds), Selenium (tuna, herring, wheat germ, wheat bran, whole grains, sesame seeds), Sulphur (fish, red peppers, garlic, onions, eggs, lean meats, cabbage, brussel sprouts, horseradish), Protein (meat, fish, poultry, soybeans, eggs, milk, whole grains), Zinc (pumpkin seeds, sunflower seeds, seafood, mushrooms, soybeans, oysters, herring, eggs, wheat germ, lean meat), E (cold-pressed oils, eggs, wheat germ, sweet potato, leafy vegetables)

ASTHMA

A (unprocessed orange vegetables and fruits), B group (whole or ground wheat, whole or ground brown rice), B6 (lean meats, whole grains, wheat germ, legumes, green leafy vegetables), B12 (fish, pork, eggs, low salt cheese, milk), Choline (egg yolk, wheat germ, soybeans, fish, legumes), Inositol (whole grains, citrus fruits, lean meat, milk, nuts, vegetables), Pangamic Acid (brown rice, sunflower seeds, pumpkin seeds, sesame seeds), Pantothenic Acid (egg yolk, legumes, whole grains, wheat germ, salmon), C (raw fruits and vegetables), D (salmon, sardines, herrings, egg yolks, organ meats), E (cold-pressed vegetable oils, eggs, wheat germ), Unsaturated Fatty Acid (vegetable oils, sunflower seeds), Calcium (skim milk, green leafy vegetables, shellfish), Manganese (whole grains, green leafy vegetables, legumes, nuts, pineapple, egg yolk)

AUTISM

B group (whole or ground wheat, whole or ground brown rice), B1 (whole grains, lean meats, fish, poultry, egg yolks), B2 (whole grains, egg yolks, legumes, nuts), B6 (lean meats, whole grains, wheat germ, legumes, green leafy vegetables), Folic Acid (dark green vegetables, root vegetables, whole grains, oysters, salmon, milk), Niacin (peanuts, rice bran, trout, salmon, rabbit, pheasant, quail), Pangamic Acid (brown rice, sunflower seeds, pumpkin seeds, sesame seeds), Pantothenic Acid (egg yolks, legumes, whole grains, wheat germ, salmon), C (raw fruits and vegetables), E (cold-pressed vegetable oils, eggs, wheat germ), Magnesium (seafood, whole grains, dark-green vegetables, nuts)

BACKACHE

B group (whole or ground wheat, whole or ground brown rice), Niacin, (peanuts, rice bran, trout, salmon, rabbit, pheasant, quail), C (raw fruits and vegetables), D (salmon, sardines, herrings, egg yolks, organ meats), E (cold-pressed vegetable oils, eggs, wheat germ), Calcium (skim milk, green leafy vegetables, shellfish), Magnesium (seafood, whole grains, dark green vegetables, nuts), Manganese (whole grains, green leafy vegetables, legumes, nuts, pineapple, egg yolk), Phosphorus (fish, lean meat, poultry, eggs, milk, nuts, whole grains), Zinc (pumpkin seeds, sunflower seeds, seafood, mushrooms, soybeans, oysters, herring, eggs, wheat germ, lean meat), Protein (meat, fish, poultry, soybeans, eggs, milk, whole grains), and filtered, detoxified rainwater

BALDNESS (ALOPECIA)

B group (whole or ground wheat, whole or ground brown rice), B1 (whole grains, lean meats, fish, poultry, egg yolks), B2 (whole grains, egg yolks, legumes, nuts), B6 (lean meats, whole grains, wheat germ, legumes, green leafy vegetables), B12 (fish, pork, eggs, low salt cheese, milk), Biotin (egg yolks, unpolished rice, whole grains, sardines, legumes), Choline (egg yolks, wheat germ, soybeans, fish, legumes), Folic Acid (dark green vegetables, root vegetables, whole grains, oysters, salmon, milk), Inositol (whole grains, citrus fruits, lean meat, milk, nuts, vegetables), Niacin (peanuts, rice bran, trout, salmon, rabbit, pheasant, quail), PABA (wheat germ, yogurt, green leafy vegetables, molasses), Pantothenic Acid (egg yolks, legumes, whole grains, wheat germ, salmon), C (raw fruits and vegetables), E (cold-pressed vegetable oils, eggs, wheat germ), Bioflavonoids (unprocessed citrus fruits, fruits, blackcurrants, buckwheat), Copper (seafood, nuts legumes, molasses, raisins), Manganese (whole grains, green leafy vegetables, legumes, nuts, pineapples, egg yolks), Potassium (lean meats, whole grains, vegetables, dried fruits, legumes, sunflower seeds), Zinc (pumpkin seeds, sunflower seeds, seafood, mushrooms, soybeans, oysters, herring, eggs, wheat germ, lean meat)

BEDSORES

A (unprocessed orange vegetables and fruits), B group (whole or ground wheat, whole or ground brown rice), B2 (whole grains, egg yolks, legumes, nuts), C (raw fruits and vegetables), D (salmon, sardines, herrings, egg yolks, organ meats), E (cold-pressed vegetable oils, eggs, wheat germ), Copper (seafood, nuts legumes, molasses, raisins), Zinc (pumpkin seeds, sunflower seeds, seafood, mushrooms, soybeans, oysters, herring, eggs, wheat germ, lean meat), Protein (meat, fish, poultry, soybeans, eggs, milk, whole grains)

BELL'S PALSY

B group (whole or ground wheat, whole or ground brown rice), B1 (including whole grains, lean meats, fish, poultry, egg yolks), C (raw fruits and vegetables), Protein (meat, fish, poultry, soybeans, eggs, milk, whole grains)

BERIBERI

B1 (whole grains, lean meats, fish, poultry, egg yolks), B group (whole or ground wheat, whole or ground brown rice), C (raw fruits and vegetables)

BODY ODOUR

B group (whole or ground wheat, whole or ground brown rice), B6 (lean meats, whole grains, wheat germ, legumes, green leafy vegetables), PABA (wheat germ, yogurt, molasses, green leafy vegetables), Magnesium (seafood, whole grains, dark green vegetables, nuts), Zinc (pumpkin seeds, sunflower seeds, seafood, mushrooms, soybeans, oysters, herring, eggs, wheat germ, lean meat)

BONE ABNORMALITIES

A (unprocessed orange vegetables and fruits), B group (whole or ground wheat, whole or ground brown rice), Pantothenic Acid (egg yolks, legumes, whole grains, wheat germ, salmon), C (raw fruits and vegetables), D (salmon, sardines, herrings, egg yolks, organ meats), E (cold-pressed vegetable oils, eggs, wheat germ), Calcium (skim milk, green leafy vegetables, shellfish), Magnesium (seafood, whole grains, dark green vegetables, nuts), Protein (meat, fish, poultry, soybeans, eggs, milk, whole grains), Unsaturated Fatty Acids (vegetable oils, sunflower seeds)

BRONCHITIS

A (unprocessed orange vegetables and fruits), C (raw fruits and vegetables), D (salmon, sardines, herrings, egg yolks, organ meats), E (cold-pressed oils, eggs, wheat germ), Unsaturated Fatty Acids (vegetable oils, sunflower seeds), Protein (lean meat, fish, poultry, soybeans, eggs, milk, whole grains e.g. whole or ground whole wheat and brown rice), and filtered, detoxified rainwater

BRUISES

B group (whole or ground wheat, whole or ground brown rice), Folic Acid (dark-green vegetables, root vegetables, whole grains, oysters, salmon, milk), C (raw fruits and vegetables), D (salmon, sardines, herrings, egg yolks, organ meats), K (green leafy vegetables, egg yolks, safflower oil, molasses, cauliflower, soybeans), Bioflavonoids (citrus fruits, fruits, black currants, buckwheat), Iron (eggs, fish, poultry, molasses, cherry juice, green leafy vegetables, dried fruits)

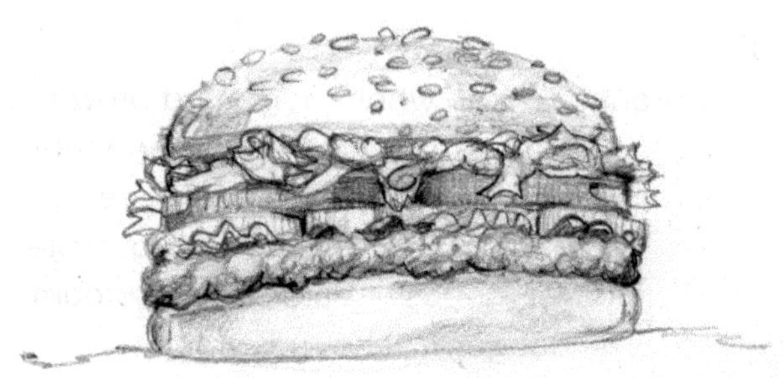

BRUXISM (TOOTH-GRINDING)

A (unprocessed orange vegetables and fruits), B1 (whole grains, lean meats, fish, poultry, egg yolks), B2 (whole grains, egg yolks, legumes, nuts), B6 (lean meats, whole grains, wheat germ, legumes, green leafy vegetables), Niacin (peanuts, rice bran, trout, salmon, rabbit, pheasant, quail), Pantothenic Acid (egg yolks, legumes, whole grains, wheat germ, salmon), C (raw fruits and vegetables), E (cold-pressed oils, eggs, wheat germ), Calcium (skim milk, green leafy vegetables, shellfish), Iodine (seafood, kelp), Protein (lean meat, fish, poultry, soybeans, eggs, milk, whole grains e.g. whole or ground whole wheat and brown rice)

BURNS

A (unprocessed orange vegetables and fruits), B group (whole or ground wheat, whole or ground brown rice), Niacin (peanuts, rice bran, trout, salmon, rabbit, pheasant, quail), PABA (wheat germ, yogurt, molasses, green leafy vegetables), Pantothenic Acid (egg yolks, legumes, whole grains, wheat germ, salmon), C (raw fruits and vegetables), D (salmon, sardines, herrings, egg yolks, organ meats), E (cold-pressed oils, eggs, wheat germ), Calcium (skim milk, green leafy vegetables, shellfish),

Iodine (seafood, kelp), Magnesium (seafood, whole grains, dark green vegetables, nuts), Unsaturated Fatty Acids (vegetable oils, sunflower seeds), Potassium (lean meats, whole grains, vegetables, dried fruits, legumes, sunflower seeds), Zinc (pumpkin seeds, sunflower seeds, seafood, mushrooms, soybeans, oysters, herring, eggs, wheat germ, lean meat), Protein (lean meat, fish, poultry, soybeans, eggs, milk, whole grains e.g. whole or ground whole wheat and brown rice), Sodium (seafood, sea salt, celery, milk products, kelp), and filtered, detoxified rainwater

BURSITIS

Bones/Muscles/Joints

A (unprocessed orange vegetables and fruits), B group (whole or ground wheat, whole or ground brown rice), B12 (fish, pork, eggs, low salt cheese, milk)

CANCER

A (unprocessed orange vegetables and fruits), B group (whole or ground wheat, whole or ground brown rice), B1 (whole grains, lean meats, fish, poultry, egg yolks), B2 (whole grains, egg yolks, legumes, nuts), B6 (lean meats, whole grains, wheat germ, legumes, green leafy vegetables), Niacin (peanuts, rice bran, trout, salmon, rabbit, pheasant, quail), Pangamic Acid (brown rice, sunflower seeds, pumpkin seeds, sesame seeds), Pantothenic Acid (egg yolks, legumes, whole grains, wheat germ, salmon), Choline (egg yolk, wheat germ, soybeans, fish, legumes), C (raw fruits and vegetables), D (salmon, sardines, herrings, egg yolks, organ meats), E (cold-pressed oils, eggs, wheat germ), K (green leafy vegetables, egg yolks, safflower oil, molasses, cauliflower, soybeans), Chromium (grapes, raisins, corn oil, clams, whole grains), Iodine (seafood, kelp), Iron (lean meats, eggs, fish, poultry, cherry juice, green leafy vegetables, dried fruits, molasses), Magnesium (seafood, whole grains, dark green vegetables, nuts), Molybdenum (legumes, whole grains, milk, dark-green vegetables), Phosphorus (fish, lean meats, poultry, eggs, milk, nuts, whole grains), Potassium (lean meats, whole grains, vegetables, legumes, sunflower seeds), Selenium (tuna, herring, wheat germ, wheat bran, whole grains, sesame seeds), Sulphur (fish, red hot peppers, garlic, onions, eggs, lean meat, cabbage, brussel sprouts, horseradish), Zinc (pumpkin seeds, sunflower seeds, seafood, mushrooms, soybeans, oysters, herring, eggs, wheat germ, lean meats), Protein (lean meat, fish, poultry, soybeans, eggs, milk, whole grains e.g. whole or ground whole wheat and brown rice), Unsaturated fatty acids (vegetable oils, sunflower seeds)

CATARACTS

A (unprocessed orange vegetables and fruits), B group (whole or ground wheat, whole or ground brown rice), B2 whole grains, egg yolks, legumes, nuts), Pantothenic Acid (egg yolks, legumes, whole grains, wheat germ, salmon), C (raw fruits and vegetables), D (salmon, sardines, herrings, egg yolks, organ meats), E (cold-pressed oils, eggs, wheat germ), Calcium (skim milk, green leafy vegetables, shellfish), Selenium (tuna, herring, wheat germ, wheat bran, whole grains, sesame seeds), Zinc (pumpkin seeds, sunflower seeds, seafood, mushrooms, soybeans, oysters, herring, eggs, wheat germ, lean meats), Protein (lean meat, fish, poultry, soybeans, eggs, milk, whole grains e.g. whole or ground whole wheat and brown rice)

CELIAC DISEASE

A (unprocessed orange vegetables and fruits), B group (gluten free ground wheat, ground brown rice), B6 (lean meats, gluten free whole grains, wheat germ, legumes, green leafy vegetables), B12 (fish, pork, eggs, low salt cheese, milk), Folic Acid (dark green vegetables, root vegetables, gluten free whole grains, oysters, salmon, milk), C (raw fruits and vegetables), D (salmon, sardines, herrings, egg yolks, organ meats), E (cold-pressed oils, eggs, wheat germ), K (green leafy vegetables, egg yolks, safflower oil, molasses, cauliflower, soybeans), Calcium (skim milk, green leafy vegetables, shellfish), Iron (lean meats, eggs, fish, poultry, cherry juice, green leafy vegetables, dried fruits, molasses), Magnesium (seafood, gluten free whole grains, dark green vegetables, nuts), Potassium (lean meats, gluten free whole grains, vegetables, dried fruits, legumes, sunflower seeds), Protein (lean meat, fish, poultry, soybeans, eggs, milk, gluten free whole grains e.g. gluten free ground whole wheat and brown rice)

CHICKEN POX

A (unprocessed orange vegetables and fruits), C (raw fruits and vegetables), Protein (lean meat, fish, poultry, soybeans, eggs, milk, whole grains e.g. whole or ground whole wheat and brown rice)

CHOLESTEROL, HIGH

B group (whole or ground wheat, whole or ground brown rice), B6 (lean meats, whole grains, wheat germ, legumes, green leafy vegetables), B12 (fish, pork, eggs, low salt cheese, milk), Biotin (egg yolks, unpolished rice, whole grains, sardines, legumes), Choline (egg yolks, wheat germ, soybeans, fish, legumes), Folic Acid (dark green leafy vegetables, root vegetables, whole grains, oysters, salmon, milk), Inositol (whole grains, citrus fruits, molasses, lean meats, milk, nuts, vegetables), PABA (wheat germ, yogurt, molasses, green leafy vegetables), Niacin (peanuts, rice bran, trout, salmon, rabbit, pheasant, quail), Pantothenic Acid (egg yolks, legumes, whole grains, wheat germ, salmon), Pangamic Acid (whole or ground brown rice, sunflower seeds, pumpkin seeds, sesame seeds), C (raw fruits and vegetables), D (salmon, sardines, herrings, egg yolks, organ meats), E (cold-pressed vegetable oils, eggs, wheat germ, sweet potato, leafy vegetables), Unsaturated Fatty Acids 1 - 2 tablespoons (cold-pressed vegetable oils, sunflower seeds), Bioflavonoids (raw citrus fruits, fruits, black currants, buckwheat), Kelp, Calcium (skim milk, green leafy vegetables, shellfish), Chromium (grapes, raisins, corn oil, clams, whole grains), Magnesium (seafood, whole grains, dark green vegetables, molasses, nuts), Manganese (whole grains, green leafy vegetables, legumes, nuts, pineapples, egg yolks), Potassium (lean meats, whole grains, vegetables, dried fruits, legumes, sunflower seeds), Selenium (tuna, herring, wheat germ, wheat bran, whole grains, sesame seeds), Vanadium (fish), Zinc (pumpkin seeds, sunflower seeds, seafood, mushrooms, soybeans, oysters, herring, eggs, wheat germ, lean meats)

CIRRHOSIS OF THE LIVER

A (unprocessed orange vegetables and fruits), B group (whole or ground wheat, whole or ground brown rice), B12 (fish, pork, eggs, low salt cheese, milk), Choline (egg yolks, wheat germ, soybeans, fish, legumes), Inositol (whole grains, citrus fruits, molasses, lean meats, milk, nuts, vegetables), Pangamic Acid (whole or ground brown rice, sunflower seeds, pumpkin seeds, sesame seeds), C (raw fruits and vegetables), D (salmon, sardines, herrings, egg yolks, organ meats), E (cold-pressed vegetable oils, eggs, wheat germ, sweet potato, leafy vegetables) Unsaturated fatty acids (cold-pressed vegetable oils, sunflower seeds), K (green leafy vegetables, egg yolks, safflower oil, molasses, cauliflower, soybeans), Magnesium (seafood, whole grains, dark green vegetables, molasses, nuts), Zinc (pumpkin seeds, sunflower seeds, seafood, mushrooms, soybeans, oysters, herring, eggs, wheat germ, lean meats), Carbohydrates (whole grains, fruits, vegetables), Protein (lean meat, fish, poultry, soybeans, eggs, milk, whole grains)

COLDS

A (unprocessed orange vegetables and fruits), B group (whole grains), B6 (lean meats, whole grains, molasses, wheat germ, legumes, green leafy vegetables), C (raw fruits and vegetables), D (salmon, sardines, herrings, egg yolks, organ meats), E (cold-pressed vegetable oils, eggs, wheat germ, sweet potato, leafy vegetables), Unsaturated fatty acids (cold-pressed vegetable oils, sunflower seeds), Bioflavonoids (raw citrus fruits, fruits, black currants, buckwheat), Calcium (skim milk, green leafy vegetables, shellfish), Zinc (pumpkin seeds, sunflower seeds, seafood, mushrooms, soybeans, oysters, herring, eggs, wheat germ, lean meats), Protein (lean meat, fish, poultry, soybeans, eggs, milk, whole grains), and filtered, detoxified rainwater

COLITIS

A (unprocessed orange vegetables and fruits), B group (whole or ground wheat, whole or ground brown rice), B6 (lean meats, whole grains, wheat germ, legumes, green leafy vegetables), Folic Acid (dark green leafy vegetables, root vegetables, whole grains, oysters, salmon, milk), Pantothenic Acid (egg yolks, legumes, whole grains, wheat germ, salmon), C, (raw fruits and vegetables), E (cold-pressed vegetable oils, eggs, wheat germ, sweet potato, leafy vegetables) Unsaturated fatty acids (cold-pressed vegetable oils, sunflower seeds), Calcium (skim milk, green leafy vegetables, shellfish), Iron (lean meats, eggs, fish, poultry, molasses, cherry juice, green leafy vegetables, dried fruits), Magnesium (seafood, whole grains, dark green vegetables, molasses, nuts), Phosphorus (fish, lean meats, poultry, eggs, milk, nuts, whole grains), Potassium (lean meats, whole grains, vegetables, dried fruits, legumes, sunflower seeds), Zinc (Pumpkin seeds, sunflower seeds, seafood, mushrooms, soybeans, oysters, herring, eggs, wheat germ, lean meats), Protein (lean meats, fish, poultry, soybeans, eggs, milk, whole grains)

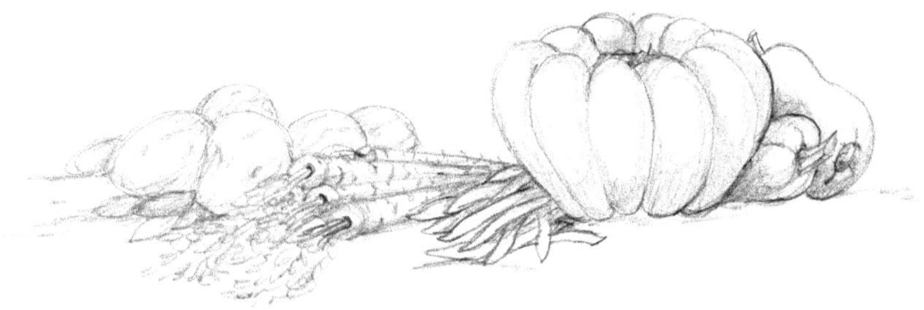

CONJUNCTIVITIS

A (unprocessed orange vegetables and fruits), B group (whole or ground wheat, whole or ground brown rice), B2 (whole grains, molasses, egg yolks, legumes, nuts), B6 (lean meats, whole grains, wheat germ, legumes, green leafy vegetables), Niacin (lean meats, poultry, fish, peanuts, milk, rice bran), C (raw fruits and vegetables), D (salmon, sardines, herrings, egg yolks, organ meats), Calcium (skim milk, green leafy vegetables, shellfish), Magnesium (seafood, whole grains, dark green vegetables, molasses, nuts), Phosphorus (fish, lean meats, poultry, eggs, milk, nuts, whole grains)

CONSTIPATION

A (unprocessed orange vegetables and fruits), B group (whole or ground wheat, whole or ground brown rice), B1 (whole grains, brown rice, lean meats, fish, poultry, egg yolks), B6 (lean meats, whole grains, wheat germ, legumes, green leafy vegetables), Choline (egg yolks, wheat germ, soybeans, fish, legumes), Inositol (whole grains, citrus fruits, lean meats, milk, nuts, vegetables), Niacin (lean meats, poultry, fish, peanuts, milk, rice bran), Pantothenic Acid (egg yolks, legumes, whole grains, wheat germ, salmon), C (raw fruits and vegetables), D (salmon, sardines, herrings, egg yolks, organ meats), E (cold-pressed vegetable oils, eggs, wheat germ, sweet potato, leafy vegetables), Unsaturated fatty acids (cold-pressed vegetable oils, sunflower seeds), Fibre (husk of wheat, raw fruits and vegetables), Calcium (skim milk, green leafy vegetables, shellfish), Magnesium (seafood, whole grains, dark green vegetables, molasses, nuts), Potassium (lean meats, whole grains, vegetables, dried fruits, legumes, sunflower seeds), Zinc (Pumpkin seeds, sunflower seeds, seafood, mushrooms, soybeans, oysters, herring, eggs, wheat germ, lean meats), Fats (vegetable oils, whole milk, nuts, seeds), and filtered, detoxified rainwater

CRETINISM

Iodine (seafood, kelp), Protein (lean meat, fish, poultry, soybeans, eggs, milk, whole grains)

CRIB DEATH

Magnesium deficiency creates a release of histamine that increases the permeability of the capillaries, allowing nutrients and oxygen to leak out and collect in sites such as the lungs. C may prevent crib death attributed to suffocation, of which the symptoms may be as slight as congested nasal passages. Crib syndrome is treated with Calcium Gluconate and C. Always seek the advice of a doctor prior to treatment. Mothers' adequate supplies of magnesium during pregnancy may prevent these conditions.

CRIME & DELINQUENCY

B1 (whole grains, brown rice, lean meats, fish, poultry, egg yolks), B6 (lean meats, whole grains, wheat germ, legumes, green leafy vegetables), Niacin (lean meats, poultry, fish, peanuts, milk, rice bran), C (raw fruits and vegetables), Zinc (Pumpkin seeds, sunflower seeds, seafood, mushrooms, soybeans, oysters, herring, eggs, wheat germ, lean meats)

CROUP

A (unprocessed orange vegetables and fruits), C (raw fruits and vegetables), Protein (lean meat, fish, poultry, soybeans, eggs, milk, whole grains e.g. whole or ground whole wheat and brown rice)

CYSTIC FIBROSIS

A (unprocessed orange vegetables and fruits), B group (whole or ground wheat, whole or ground brown rice), B2 (whole grains, egg yolks, legumes, nuts), B6 (lean meats, whole grains, wheat germ, legumes, molasses, green leafy vegetables), Pantothenic Acid (egg yolks, legumes, whole grains, wheat germ, salmon), C (raw fruits and vegetables), D (salmon, sardines, herrings, egg yolks, organ meats), E (cold-pressed vegetable oils, eggs, wheat germ, sweet potato, leafy vegetables), K (green leafy vegetables, egg yolks, safflower oil, molasses, cauliflower, soybeans), Copper (seafood, nuts, legumes, molasses, raisins), Selenium (tuna, herring, wheat germ, wheat bran, whole grains, sesame seeds), Sodium (sea salt, with no added anti-caking agent – 554, E554), Zinc (Pumpkin seeds, sunflower seeds, seafood, mushrooms, soybeans, oysters, herring, eggs, wheat germ, lean meats), Protein (lean meat, fish, poultry, soybeans, eggs, milk, whole grains e.g. whole or ground whole wheat and brown rice)

CYSTITIS (BLADDER INFECTION)

A (unprocessed orange vegetables and fruits), B group (whole or ground wheat, whole or ground brown rice), B6 (lean meats, whole grains, wheat germ, legumes, green leafy vegetables) Pantothenic Acid (including egg yolks, legumes, whole grains, wheat germ, salmon), C (raw fruits and vegetables), D (salmon, sardines, herrings, egg yolks, organ meats), E (cold-pressed vegetable oils, eggs, wheat germ, sweet potato, leafy vegetables), Zinc (pumpkin seeds, sunflower seeds, seafood, mushrooms, soybeans, oysters, herring, eggs, wheat germ, lean meats), and filtered, detoxified rainwater

DANDRUFF

A (unprocessed orange vegetables and fruits), B group (whole or ground wheat, whole or ground brown rice), B6 (lean meats, whole grains, wheat germ, legumes, molasses, green leafy vegetables), C (raw fruits and vegetables), E (cold-pressed vegetable oils, eggs, wheat germ, sweet potato, leafy vegetables), Unsaturated fatty acids (cold-pressed vegetable oils, sunflower seeds), Selenium (tuna, herring, wheat germ, wheat bran, whole grains, sesame seeds), Zinc (pumpkin seeds, sunflower seeds, seafood, mushrooms, soybeans, oysters, herring, eggs, wheat germ, lean meats), and filtered, detoxified rainwater

DEAFNESS

A (unprocessed orange vegetables and fruits), B group (whole grains i.e. whole or ground wheat, whole or ground brown rice), C (raw fruits and vegetables), E (cold-pressed vegetable oils, eggs, wheat germ), Zinc (pumpkin seeds, sunflower seeds, seafood, mushrooms, soybeans, oysters, herring, egg, wheat germ, lean meats)

DEPRESSION

"I am centred and calm and balanced. The Universe does approve of me. I trust my intuition and that little voice inside of me. I go beyond other people's fears and create my own life." Repeat until this begins to feel true for you.

DERMATITIS

A (unprocessed orange vegetables and fruits), B group (whole grains i.e. whole or ground wheat, whole or ground brown rice), B2 (whole grains, egg yolks, legumes, nuts), B6 (lean meats, whole grains, wheat germ, legumes, molasses, green leafy vegetables), Biotin (egg yolks, unpolished rice, whole grains, sardines, legumes), Niacin (lean meats, poultry, fish, peanuts, milk, rice bran), D (salmon, sardines, herrings, egg yolks, organ meats), Unsaturated fatty acids (cold-pressed vegetable oils, sunflower seeds), Potassium (Lean meats, whole grains, vegetables, dried fruits, legumes, sunflower seeds), Sulphur (fish, red hot peppers, garlic, onions, eggs, lean meats, cabbage, brussel sprouts, horseradish), Zinc (pumpkin seeds, sunflower seeds, seafood, mushrooms, soybeans, oysters, herring, egg, wheat germ, lean meats), Protein (lean meat, fish, poultry, soybeans, eggs, milk, whole grains e.g. whole or ground whole wheat and brown rice), and filtered, detoxified rainwater

DIABETES

Chromium (grapes, raisins, corn oil, clams, whole grains), A (unprocessed orange vegetables and fruits), B Group (whole grains i.e. whole or ground wheat, whole or ground brown rice), B1 (sunflower seeds, pistachios, quail, pork, whole grains, molasses, brown rice, lean meats, fish, poultry, egg yolks), B2 (almonds, wild rice, venison), B6 (brown rice, pinto beans, trout, sunflower seeds), B12 (oysters, herring, crab, trout, mackerel, clams, bass, flounder/sole, salmon, scallops, trout, pork, eggs, milk), Inositol (

citrus fruits, milk, nuts, vegetables, whole grains), Niacin (peanuts, lean meats, poultry, fish, milk, rice bran), Pantothenic Acid (egg yolk, legumes, whole grains, wheat germ, salmon), Pangamic Acid, C (brown rice, sunflower seeds, pumpkin seeds, sesame seeds), D (salmon, sardines, herrings, egg yolks, organ meats), E (cold-pressed vegetable oils, egg, wheat germ, sweet potato, leaf vegetables), Unsaturated fatty acids 2 tablespoons (vegetable oils, sunflower seeds), Calcium (milk, almonds, green leafy vegetables, shellfish), Iron (lean meats, fish, poultry, cherry juice, green leafy vegetables, dried fruits), Magnesium (seafood, whole grains, dark green vegetables, nuts), Manganese (whole grains, green leafy vegetables, legumes, nuts, pineapple, egg yolk), Potassium (vegetables, whole grains, lean meat, legumes, sunflower seeds, dried fruits), Zinc (pumpkin seeds, sunflower seeds, seafood, mushrooms, soybeans, oysters, herring, eggs, wheat germ, lean meat), Protein (lean meat, fish, poultry, soybean, eggs, milk, whole grains)

DIARRHOEA

Bowel: A (unprocessed orange vegetables and fruits), B group (whole grains i.e. whole or ground wheat, whole or ground brown rice), B1 (whole grains, molasses, brown rice, lean meats, fish, poultry, egg yolks, sunflower seeds, pistachios, quail, pork), B2 (almonds, wild rice, venison), B6 (brown rice, pinto beans, trout, sunflower seeds), Folic Acid (dark green leafy vegetables, root vegetables, whole grains, oysters, salmon, milk), Niacin (peanuts, lean meats, poultry, fish, milk, rice bran), Pantothenic Acid (egg yolk, legumes, whole grains, wheat germ, salmon), C (raw fruits and vegetables)

Cells: Unsaturated fatty acids (cold-pressed vegetable oils, sunflower seeds), Calcium (milk, almonds, green leafy vegetables, shellfish), Chlorine (seafood, sea salt, lean meats, ripe olives, rye flour), Iron (lean meats, eggs, fish, poultry, molasses, cherry juice, green leafy vegetables, dried fruits), Magnesium (seafood, whole grains, dark green vegetables, nuts), Potassium (vegetables, whole grains, lean meat, legumes, sunflower seeds, dried fruits), Sodium (seafood, sea salt, celery, milk products, kelp), Fibre (husk of wheat, raw fruits and vegetables), Protein (lean meat, fish, poultry, soybean, eggs, milk, whole grains), and filtered, detoxified rainwater

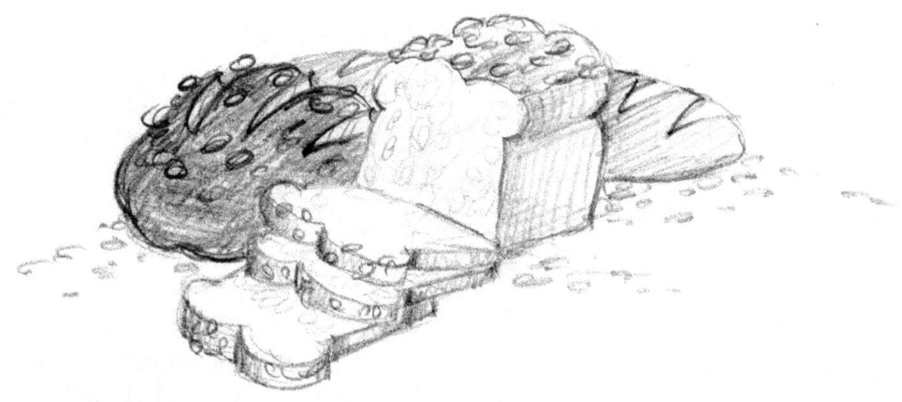

DIVERTICULITIS

B group (whole grains i.e. whole or ground wheat, whole or ground brown rice), Folic Acid (dark green leafy vegetables, root vegetables, whole grains, oysters, salmon, milk), C (raw fruits and vegetables), Fibre (husks of wheat, fruits, vegetables), plain natural yogurt, and filtered, detoxified rainwater

DIZZINESS/VERTIGO

B group (whole grains i.e. whole or ground wheat, whole or ground brown rice), B1 (whole grains, molasses, brown rice, lean meats, fish, poultry, egg yolks, sunflower seeds, pistachios, quail, pork), B2 (almonds, wild rice, venison), B6 (brown rice, pinto beans, trout, sunflower seeds), B12 (oysters, herring, crab, trout, mackerel, clams, bass, flounder, sole, salmon, scallops, trout, pork, eggs, milk), Choline (egg yolks, wheat germ, soybeans, fish, legumes), Inositol (whole grains, citrus fruits, lean meats, milk, nuts, vegetables), Niacin (lean meats, poultry, fish, peanuts, milk, rice bran), C (raw fruits and vegetables), E (cold-pressed vegetable oils, egg, wheat germ, sweet potato, leaf vegetables), Calcium (milk, almonds, green leafy vegetables, shellfish)

DRUG ABUSE OR DEPENDENCY

C (raw fruits and vegetables), Calcium (milk, almonds, green leafy vegetables, shellfish), Potassium (vegetables, whole grains, lean meat, legumes, sunflower seeds, dried fruits), Magnesium (seafood, whole grains, dark green vegetables, nuts)

* Large doses of Vitamin C have been successfully used to cure heroin, methadone, and barbiturate addiction. Heroin use increases body acid and causes the depletion of potassium and calcium. Ref: "Nutrition Almanac" by John D. Kirschmann, (1990), Available: McGraw-Hill

EAR INFECTION

A (unprocessed orange vegetables and fruits), B group (whole grains i.e. whole or ground wheat, whole or ground brown rice), C (raw fruits and vegetables), Protein (lean meat, fish, poultry, soybean, eggs, milk, whole grains)

ECZEMA

A (unprocessed orange vegetables and fruits), B group (whole grains i.e. whole or ground wheat, whole or ground brown rice), B2 (almonds, wild rice, venison), B6 (brown rice, pinto beans, trout, sunflower seeds), Biotin (egg yolks, unpolished rice, whole grains, sardines, legumes), Choline (egg yolks, wheat germ, soybeans, fish, legumes), Inositol (whole grains, citrus fruits, lean meats, milk, nuts, vegetables), PABA (wheat germ, yogurt, molasses, green leafy vegetables), C (raw fruits and vegetables), D (salmon, sardines, herrings, egg yolks, organ meats), Unsaturated fatty acids 1 - 3 tablespoons (cold-pressed vegetable oils, sunflower seeds), Magnesium (seafood, whole grains, dark green vegetables, nuts), Sulphur (fish, red hot peppers, garlic, onions, eggs, lean meats, cabbage, brussel sprouts, horseradish), Zinc (pumpkin seeds, sunflower seeds, seafood, mushrooms, soybeans, oysters, herring, eggs, wheat germ, lean meats)

EMPHYSEMA

A (unprocessed orange vegetables and fruits), B group (whole grains i.e. whole or ground wheat, whole or ground brown rice), Folic Acid (dark green leafy vegetables, root vegetables, whole grains, oysters, salmon, milk), Pangamic Acid (brown rice, sunflower seeds, pumpkin seeds, sesame seeds), C (raw fruits and vegetables), D (salmon, sardines, herrings, egg yolks, organ meats), E (cold-pressed vegetable oils, egg, wheat germ, sweet potato, leaf vegetables), Protein (lean meat, fish, poultry, soybean, eggs, milk, whole grains)

ENVIRONMENTAL POLLUTION

A (unprocessed orange vegetables and fruits), B group (whole grains i.e. whole or ground wheat, whole or ground brown rice), B1 (whole grains, molasses, brown rice, lean meats, fish, poultry, egg yolks, sunflower seeds, pistachios, quail, pork), B6 (brown rice, pinto beans, trout, sunflower seeds), Niacin (lean meats, poultry, fish, peanuts, milk, rice bran), PABA (wheat germ, yogurt, molasses, green leafy vegetables), Pantothenic Acid (egg yolks, legumes, whole grains, wheat germ, salmon), C (raw fruits and vegetables), E (cold-pressed vegetable oils, egg, wheat germ, sweet potato, leaf vegetables), Calcium (milk, almonds, green leafy vegetables, shellfish), Selenium (tuna, herring, wheat germ, wheat bran, whole grains, sesame seeds), Zinc (pumpkin seeds, sunflower seeds, seafood, mushrooms, soybeans, oysters, herring, eggs, wheat germ, lean meats), Protein (lean meat, fish, poultry, soybean, eggs, milk, whole grains)

EPILEPSY

A (unprocessed orange vegetables and fruits), B group (whole grains i.e. whole or ground wheat, whole or ground brown rice), B6 (brown rice, pinto beans, trout, sunflower seeds), B12 (fish, pork, eggs, milk, low salt cheese), Folic Acid (including dark green leafy vegetables, root vegetables, whole grains, oysters, salmon, milk), B3 (lean meats, poultry, fish, peanuts, milk, rice bran), Pangamic Acid (brown rice, sunflower seeds, pumpkin seeds, sesame seeds), C (raw fruits and vegetables), D (salmon, sardines, herrings, egg yolks, organ meats), E (cold-pressed vegetable oils, egg, wheat germ, sweet potato, leaf vegetables), Calcium (milk, almonds, green leafy vegetables, shellfish), Magnesium (seafood, whole grains, dark green vegetables, nuts), Manganese (whole grains, dark-green vegetables, molasses, nuts)

EYE DISORDERS

Dry Eyelids, Tired Eyes, Sensitivity to Light Variations, Susceptibility to Eye Infections, Ulcerations, Irreversible Blindness: A (unprocessed orange vegetables and fruits), and filtered, detoxified rainwater

Watering Eyes, Itching, Burning, Light Sensitivity, Bloodshot Eyes, Paralysed Eye Muscles: B group (whole grains i.e. whole or ground wheat, whole or ground brown rice), and filtered, detoxified rainwater

Spots Floating In Front of the Eyes, Colour Disturbance, Halos Around Lights or Objects, Inability To See Part of an Image or Printed Page: B2 (almonds, wild rice, venison, whole grains, egg yolks, blackstrap molasses, legumes, nuts)

Prevent Tissue Hemorrhaging and Capillary Fragility, Infections: C (raw fruits and vegetables), Rutin (grapes, plums, blackcurrants, apricots, buckwheat, cherries, blackberries, rose hips)

Weak Eye Muscles, Blurred Vision, Double Vision, Crossed Eyes, Detached Retina, Retinal Hemorrhage, Protruding Eyes: E (cold-pressed vegetable oils, egg, wheat germ, sweet potato, leaf vegetables), A (unprocessed orange vegetables and fruits), C (raw fruits and vegetables), B group (whole grains i.e. whole or ground wheat, whole or ground brown rice)

AMBLYOPIA

B1 (whole grains, molasses, brown rice, lean meats, fish, poultry, egg yolks, sunflower seeds, pistachios, quail, pork)

BITOT'S SPOT

A (unprocessed orange vegetables and fruits), Protein (lean meat, fish, poultry, soybeans, eggs, milk, whole grains)

CORNEAL ULCERS

B2 (almonds, wild rice, venison, whole grains, molasses, egg yolks, legumes, nuts), B6 (brown rice, pinto beans, trout, sunflower seeds, whole grains, wheat germ, legumes, green leafy vegetables), Pantothenic Acid (egg yolks, legumes, whole grains, wheat germ, salmon), C (raw fruits and vegetables), Protein (lean meat, fish, poultry, soybeans, eggs, milk, whole grains)

NEARSIGHTEDNESS

Calcium, B2 (almonds, wild rice, venison, whole grains, molasses, egg yolks, legumes, nuts), C (raw fruits and vegetables), D (salmon, sardines, herrings, egg yolks, organ meats), E (cold-pressed vegetable oils, egg, wheat germ, sweet potato, leaf vegetables), Pantothenic Acid (egg yolks, legumes, whole grains, wheat germ, salmon), Protein (lean meat, fish, poultry, soybeans, eggs, milk, whole grains), Unsaturated fatty acids (vegetable oils, sunflower seeds)

NIGHT BLINDNESS

A (unprocessed orange vegetables and fruits), B2 (almonds, wild rice, venison, whole grains, egg yolks, molasses, legumes, nuts), Niacin (peanuts, fish, lean meats, poultry, milk, rice bran), B1 (whole grains, brown rice, egg yolks, fish, molasses, lean meats, poultry) and Zinc (pumpkin seeds, sunflower seeds, seafood, mushrooms, soybeans, oysters, herring, eggs, wheat germ, lean meats)

RETINITIS PIGMENTOSA

A (unprocessed orange vegetables and fruits), Unsaturated fatty acids (vegetable oils, sunflower seeds), E (cold-pressed vegetable oils, egg, wheat germ, sweet potato, leaf vegetables)

GOOD EYE HEALTH

A (unprocessed orange vegetables and fruits), B group (whole grains i.e. whole or ground wheat, whole or ground brown rice), C (raw fruits and vegetables), E (cold-pressed vegetable oils, egg, wheat germ, sweet potato, leaf vegetables), Protein (lean meat, fish, poultry, soybeans, eggs, milk, whole grains)

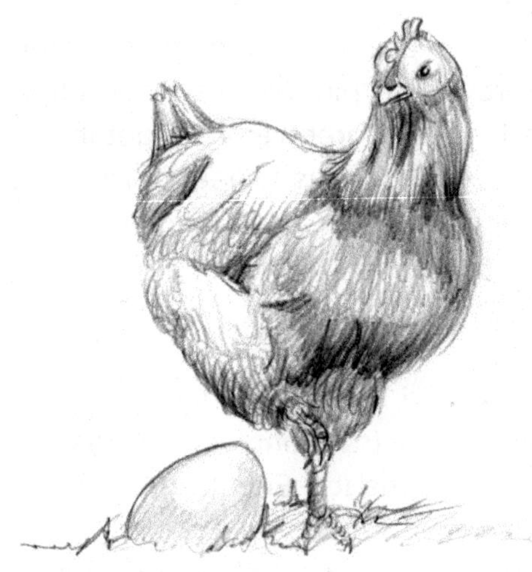

EYES

A (unprocessed orange vegetables and fruits), B group (whole grains i.e. whole or ground wheat, whole or ground brown rice), B1 (whole grains, molasses, brown rice, lean meats, fish, poultry, egg yolks, sunflower seeds, pistachios, quail, pork), B2 (almonds, wild rice, venison, whole grains, molasses, egg yolks, legumes, nuts), B6 (brown rice, pinto beans, trout, sunflower seeds, whole grains, wheat germ, legumes, green leafy vegetables), Niacin (peanuts, fish, lean meats, poultry, milk, rice bran), Pantothenic Acid (egg yolks, legumes, whole grains, wheat germ, salmon), C (raw fruits and vegetables), Bioflavonoids (citrus fruits, fruits, blackcurrants, buckwheat), D (salmon, sardines, herrings, egg yolks, organ meats), E (cold-pressed vegetable oils, egg, wheat germ, sweet potato, leaf vegetables), Calcium (milk, almonds, green leafy vegetables, shellfish), Magnesium (seafood, whole grains, dark green vegetables, nuts), Zinc (pumpkin seeds, sunflower seeds, seafood, mushrooms, soybeans, oysters, herring, eggs, wheat germ, lean meats), Protein (lean meat, fish, poultry, soybeans, eggs, milk, whole grains), Unsaturated fatty acids (vegetable oils, sunflower seeds), and filtered, detoxified rainwater

FATIGUE

A (unprocessed orange vegetables and fruits), B group (whole grains i.e. whole or ground wheat, whole or ground brown rice), Folic Acid (dark green leafy vegetables, root vegetables, whole grains, oysters, salmon, milk), C (raw fruits and vegetables), D (salmon, sardines, herrings, egg yolks, organ meats), Iron (lean meats, fish, poultry, cherry juice, green leafy vegetables, dried fruits), Magnesium (seafood, whole grains, dark green vegetables, nuts), Manganese (whole grains, green leafy vegetables, legumes, nuts, pineapple, egg yolks, lima beans, sunflower seeds, tapioca, blackberries), Potassium (lean meats, whole grains, vegetables, dried fruits, legumes, sunflower seeds, avocados, cantaloupes - rockmelons, plantains), Fibre (bran)

FATIGUE, CHRONIC

**"I am enthusiastic about life and filled with energy and enthusiasm."* Repeat until this begins to feel true for you (Hay, 1987).

FEVER

A (unprocessed orange vegetables and fruits), B group (whole grains i.e. whole or ground wheat, whole or ground brown rice), B1 (whole grains, molasses, brown rice, lean meats, fish, poultry, egg yolks, sunflower seeds, pistachios, quail, pork), C (raw fruits and vegetables), D (salmon, sardines, herrings, egg yolks, organ meats), Calcium (milk, almonds, green leafy vegetables, shellfish), Phosphorus (nuts, whole grains, fish, lean meats, poultry, eggs, milk, garbanzos) Potassium (lean meats, whole grains, vegetables, dried fruits, legumes, sunflower seeds, avocados, cantaloupes, plantains), Sodium (kelp), Protein (lean meat, fish, poultry, soybeans, eggs, milk, whole grains)

FLATULENCE (INTESTINAL GAS)

B group (whole grains i.e. whole or ground wheat, whole or ground brown rice), Pantothenic Acid (egg yolks, legumes, whole grains, wheat germ, salmon), plain natural yogurt

FLU

A (unprocessed orange vegetables and fruits), B group (whole grains i.e. whole or ground wheat, whole or ground brown rice), B1 (whole grains, molasses, brown rice, lean meats, fish, poultry, egg yolks, sunflower seeds, pistachios, quail, pork), B2 (almonds, wild rice, venison, whole grains, molasses, egg yolks, legumes, nuts), B6 (brown rice, pinto beans, trout, sunflower seeds, whole grains, wheat germ, legumes, green leafy vegetables), C (raw fruits and vegetables), Niacin (peanuts, fish, lean meats, poultry, milk, rice bran), Pantothenic Acid (egg yolks, legumes, whole grains, wheat germ, salmon), Potassium (lean meats, whole grains, vegetables, dried fruits, legumes, sunflower seeds, avocados, cantaloupes, plantains), Protein (lean meat, fish, poultry, soybeans, eggs, milk, whole grains)

FLUID RETENTION

B group (whole grains i.e. whole or ground wheat, whole or ground brown rice), B1 (whole grains, molasses, brown rice, fish, lean meats, poultry, egg yolks, sunflower seeds, pistachios, quail, pork), B6 (brown rice, pinto beans, trout, sunflower seeds), Pantothenic Acid (salmon, egg yolks, legumes, whole grains, wheat germ), C (raw fruits and vegetables),

D (salmon, sardines, herrings, egg yolks, organ meats), E (cold-pressed vegetable oils, egg, wheat germ, sweet potato, leaf vegetables), Calcium (milk, almonds, green leafy vegetables, shellfish), Copper (seafood, nuts, legumes, molasses, raisins), Potassium (whole grains, vegetables, dried fruits, legumes, sunflower seeds, lean meats), Protein (fish, lean meat, poultry, soybean, eggs, milk, whole grains)

Low Sodium Retention due to an under-active thyroid: Phosphorous (fish, lean meats, poultry, eggs, milk, nuts, whole grains), Iodine (seafood, kelp) Retention due to pre-menstruation: Calcium (milk, almonds, green leafy vegetables, shellfish), Zinc (pumpkin seeds, sunflower seeds, seafood, mushrooms, soybeans, oysters, herring, eggs, wheat germ, lean meats), Magnesium (seafood, whole grains, dark green vegetables, nuts), D (salmon, sardines, herrings, egg yolks, organ meats)

FRACTURE (BROKEN BONE)

A (unprocessed orange vegetables and fruits), Pantothenic Acid (egg yolks, legumes, whole grains, wheat germ, salmon), C (raw fruits and vegetables), D (salmon, sardines, herrings, egg yolks, organ meats), Calcium (milk, almonds, green leafy vegetables, shellfish), Magnesium (seafood, whole grains, dark green vegetables, nuts), Phosphorus (fish, lean meats, poultry, eggs, milk, nuts, whole grains), Potassium (lean meats, whole grains, vegetables, dried fruits, legumes, sunflower seeds, avocados, cantaloupes, plantains), Protein (whole grains, soybeans, eggs, milk, lean meats, fish, poultry), Silicon (plant fibre, hard drinking water)

GALLBLADDER DISORDERS

A (unprocessed orange vegetables and fruits), B group (whole grains i.e. whole or ground wheat, whole or ground brown rice), C (raw fruits and vegetables), D (salmon, sardines, herrings, egg yolks, organ meats), E (cold-pressed vegetable oils, egg, wheat germ, sweet potato, leaf vegetables), plain natural yogurt

GALLSTONES

A (unprocessed orange vegetables and fruits), B group (whole grains i.e. whole or ground wheat, whole or ground brown rice), C (raw fruits and vegetables), D (salmon, sardines, herrings, egg yolks, organ meats), E (cold-pressed vegetable oils, egg, wheat germ, sweet potato, leaf vegetables), K (green leafy vegetables, egg yolks, safflower oil, molasses, cauliflower, soybeans), Bran

GASTRITIS

A (unprocessed orange vegetables and fruits), B group (whole grains i.e. whole or ground wheat, whole or ground brown rice), B6 (brown rice, pinto beans, trout, sunflower seeds, whole grains, wheat germ, legumes, green leafy vegetables, B12, Folic Acid (dark green leafy vegetables, root vegetables, whole grains, oysters, salmon, milk), Inositol (whole grains, citrus fruits, molasses, lean meats, milk, nuts, vegetables), Pantothenic Acid (egg yolks, legumes, whole grains, wheat germ, salmon), C (raw fruits and vegetables), D (salmon, sardines, herrings, egg yolks, organ meats), E (cold-pressed vegetable oils, egg, wheat germ, sweet potato, leaf vegetables), Calcium (milk, almonds, green leafy vegetables, shellfish), Iron (lean meats, eggs, fish, poultry, molasses, cherry juice, green leafy vegetables, dried fruits)

GLAUCOMA

A (unprocessed orange vegetables and fruits), B group (whole grains i.e. whole or ground wheat, whole or ground brown rice), B2 (almonds, wild rice, venison, whole grains, molasses, egg yolks, legumes, nuts), Choline (egg yolks, wheat germ, soybeans, fish, legumes), Inositol (whole grains, citrus fruits, molasses, lean meats, milk, nuts, vegetables), C (raw fruits and vegetables), D (salmon, sardines, herrings, egg yolks, organ meats), Bioflavonoids (citrus fruits, fruits, blackcurrants, buckwheat)

GOITRE

A (unprocessed orange vegetables and fruits), B group (whole grains i.e. whole or ground wheat, whole or ground brown rice), B6 (brown rice, pinto beans, trout, sunflower seeds, whole grains, wheat germ, legumes, green leafy vegetables), Choline (egg yolks, wheat germ, soybeans, fish, legumes), C (raw fruits and vegetables), E (cold-pressed vegetable oils, egg, wheat germ, sweet potato, leaf vegetables), Calcium (milk, almonds, green leafy vegetables, shellfish), Iodine (seafood, kelp), Protein (lean meat, fish, poultry, soybeans, eggs, milk, whole grains)

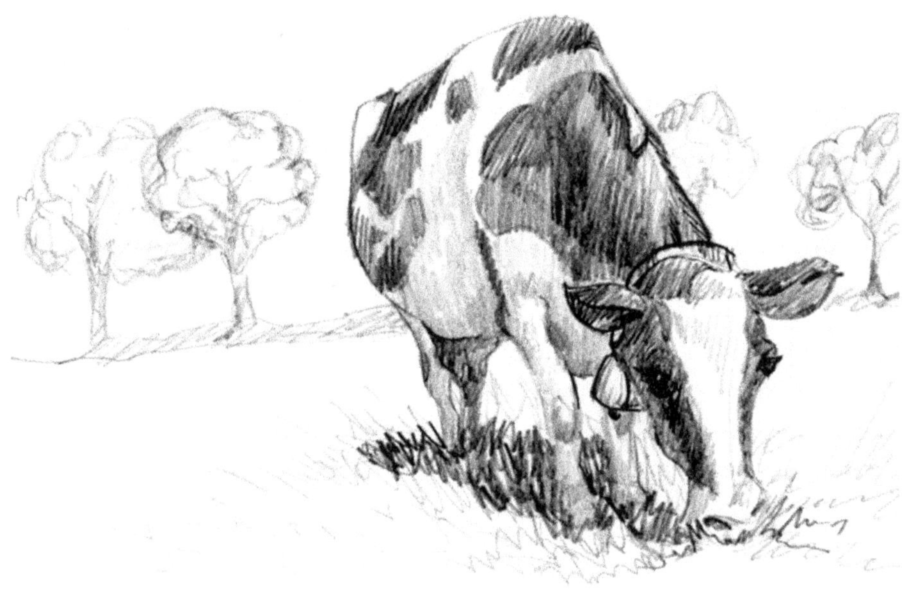

GOUT

A (unprocessed orange vegetables and fruits), B group (whole grains i.e. whole or ground wheat, whole or ground brown rice), B1 (whole grains, molasses, brown rice, fish, lean meats, poultry, egg yolks, sunflower seeds, pistachios, quail, pork), Pantothenic Acid (egg yolks, legumes, whole grains, wheat germ, salmon), C (raw fruits and vegetables), E (cold-pressed vegetable oils, egg, wheat germ, sweet potato, leaf vegetables), Calcium (milk, almonds, green leafy vegetables, shellfish), Iron (lean meats, fish, poultry, cherry juice, green leafy vegetables, dried fruits), Magnesium (seafood, whole grains, dark green vegetables, nuts), Phosphorus (fish, lean meats, poultry, eggs, milk, nuts, whole grains) Potassium (lean meats, whole grains, vegetables, dried fruits, legumes, sunflower seeds, avocados, cantaloupes, plantains), Complete Protein (lean meat, fish, poultry, soybeans, eggs, milk, whole grains)

HAIR PROBLEMS

A (unprocessed orange vegetables and fruits), B group (whole grains i.e. whole or ground wheat, whole or ground brown rice), B6 (brown rice, pinto beans, trout, sunflower seeds, whole grains, wheat germ, legumes, green leafy vegetables), Biotin (egg yolks, unpolished rice, whole grains, sardines, legumes) Folic Acid (dark green leafy vegetables, root vegetables, whole grains, oysters, salmon, milk), Inositol (whole grains, citrus fruits, molasses, lean meats, milk, nuts, vegetables), PABA (wheat germ, plain, natural yogurt, molasses, green leafy vegetables), Pantothenic Acid (egg yolks, legumes, whole grains, wheat germ, salmon), C (raw fruits and vegetables), Copper (seafood, nuts, legumes, molasses, raisins), Iodine (seafood, kelp), Magnesium (seafood, whole grains, dark green vegetables, nuts), Sulphur (fish, red hot peppers, garlic, onions, eggs, lean meats, cabbage, brussel sprouts, horseradish), Zinc (pumpkin seeds, sunflower seeds, seafood, mushrooms, soybeans, oysters, herring, eggs, wheat germ, lean meats), Protein (lean meat, fish, poultry, soybeans, eggs, milk, whole grains)

HALITOSIS

A (unprocessed orange vegetables and fruits), B group (whole grains i.e. whole or ground wheat, whole or ground brown rice), B6 (brown rice, pinto beans, trout, sunflower seeds, whole grains, wheat germ, legumes, green leafy vegetables), Niacin (peanuts, lean meats, fish, poultry, milk, rice bran), PABA (wheat germ, plain natural yogurt, molasses, green leafy vegetables), C (raw fruits and vegetables), Magnesium (seafood, whole grains, dark green vegetables, nuts), Zinc (pumpkin seeds, sunflower seeds, seafood, mushrooms, soybeans, oysters, herring, eggs, wheat germ, lean meats), plain natural yogurt

HAY FEVER (ALLERGIC RHINITIS)

A (unprocessed orange vegetables and fruits), B group (whole grains i.e. whole or ground wheat, whole or ground brown rice), C (raw fruits and vegetables), E (cold-pressed vegetable oils, egg, wheat germ, sweet potato, leaf vegetables)

HEADACHE

A (unprocessed orange vegetables and fruits), B group (whole grains i.e. whole or ground wheat, whole or ground brown rice), B1 (whole grains, molasses, brown rice, fish, lean meats, poultry, egg yolks, sunflower seeds, pistachios, quail, pork), B2 (almonds, wild rice, venison, whole grains, molasses, egg yolks, legumes, nuts), B6 (brown rice, pinto beans, trout, sunflower seeds, whole grains, wheat germ, legumes, green leafy vegetables), Niacin (peanuts, fish, lean meats, poultry, milk, rice bran), Pangamic Acid (brown rice, sunflower seeds, pumpkin seeds, sesame seeds), Pantothenic Acid (egg yolks, legumes, whole grains, wheat germ, salmon), C (raw fruits and vegetables), D (salmon, sardines, herrings, egg yolks, organ meats), E (cold-pressed vegetable oils, egg, wheat germ, sweet potato, leaf vegetables), Calcium (milk, almonds, green leafy vegetables, shellfish), Iron (lean meats, fish, poultry, cherry juice, green leafy vegetables, dried fruits), Magnesium (seafood, whole grains, dark green vegetables, nuts), Potassium (lean meats, whole grains, vegetables, dried fruits, legumes, sunflower seeds, avocados, cantaloupes, plantains), Zinc (pumpkin seeds, sunflower seeds, seafood, mushrooms, soybeans, oysters, herring, eggs, wheat germ, lean meats), Tryptophan (bananas, milk), natural yogurt

HEART DISEASE

A (unprocessed orange vegetables and fruits), B group (whole grains i.e. whole or ground wheat, whole or ground brown rice), B1 (whole grains, molasses, brown rice, fish, lean meats, poultry, egg yolks, sunflower seeds, pistachios, quail, pork), B6 (brown rice, pinto beans, trout, sunflower seeds, whole grains, wheat germ, legumes, green leafy vegetables), Choline (egg yolks, wheat germ, whole grains, legumes), Folic Acid (dark green leafy vegetables, root vegetables, whole grains, oysters, salmon, milk), Inositol (whole grains, citrus fruits, molasses, lean meats, milk, nuts, vegetables), Niacin (peanuts, fish, lean meats, poultry, milk, rice bran), D (salmon, sardines, herrings, egg yolks, organ meats), E (cold-pressed vegetable oils, egg, wheat germ, sweet potato, leaf vegetables), Calcium (milk, almonds, green leafy vegetables, shellfish), Chromium (grapes, raisins, corn oil, clams, whole grains), Copper (seafood, nuts, legumes, molasses, raisins), Iodine (seafood, kelp), Magnesium (seafood, whole grains, dark green vegetables, nuts), Manganese (whole grains, green leafy vegetables, legumes, nuts, pineapple, egg yolks, lima beans, sunflower seeds, tapioca, blackberries), Phosphorus regulated carefully (whole grains, nuts, milk, eggs, fish, lean meats, poultry), Selenium (tuna, herring, wheat germ, wheat bran, whole grains, sesame seeds),

Zinc (pumpkin seeds, sunflower seeds, seafood, mushrooms, soybeans, oysters, herring, eggs, wheat germ, lean meats), Protein (whole grains, milk, eggs, soybeans, fish, lean meats, poultry), Unsaturated fatty acids (vegetable oils, sunflower seeds)

HEMOLYTIC ANAEMIA

E (wheat germ, egg, sweet potato, cold-pressed vegetable oils, leaf vegetables, cucumber), Folic Acid (dark-green leafy vegetables, root vegetables, whole grains, oysters, salmon, milk),

HEMOPHILIA

Niacin (peanuts, fish, lean meats, poultry, milk, rice bran), C (raw fruits and vegetables), Bioflavonoids (citrus fruits, fruits, black currants, buckwheat), E (cold-pressed vegetable oils, egg, wheat germ, sweet potato, leaf vegetables), Calcium (milk, almonds, green leafy vegetables, shellfish), plain natural yoghurt

HEMORRHOIDS (PILES)

A (unprocessed orange vegetables and fruits), B group (whole grains i.e. whole or ground wheat, whole or ground brown rice), B6 (brown rice, pinto beans, trout, sunflower seeds, whole grains, wheat germ, legumes, green leafy vegetables), C (raw fruits and vegetables), E (cold-pressed vegetable oils, egg, wheat germ, sweet potato, leaf vegetables), Bioflavonoids (citrus fruits, fruits, blackcurrants, buckwheat), Calcium (milk, almonds, green leafy vegetables, shellfish), Fluids: filtered, detoxified rainwater and herbal teas, Fibre (bran)

HEPATITIS

A (unprocessed orange vegetables and fruits), B group (whole grains i.e. whole or ground wheat, whole or ground brown rice), B6 (brown rice, pinto beans, trout, sunflower seeds, whole grains, wheat germ, legumes, green leafy vegetables), Pangamic Acid (brown rice, sunflower seeds, pumpkin seeds, sesame seeds), Pantothenic Acid (egg yolks, legumes, whole grains, wheat germ, salmon), C (raw fruits and vegetables), E (cold-pressed vegetable oils, egg, wheat germ, sweet potato, leaf vegetables), Unsaturated fatty acids (vegetable oils, sunflower seeds), Protein (lean meat, fish, poultry, soybeans, eggs, milk, whole grains),

Zinc (pumpkin seeds, sunflower seeds, seafood, mushrooms, soybeans, oysters, herring, eggs, wheat germ, lean meats), Fluids: filtered, detoxified rainwater and herbal teas

HERPES SIMPLEX I and II

B group (whole grains i.e. whole or ground wheat, whole or ground brown rice), C (raw fruits and vegetables), E (cold-pressed vegetable oils, egg, wheat germ, sweet potato, leaf vegetables), Zinc (pumpkin seeds, sunflower seeds, seafood, mushrooms, soybeans, oysters, herring, eggs, wheat germ, lean meats), Lysine (lean beef, veal, pork)

HYPERACTIVITY

B1 (whole grains, molasses, brown rice, fish, lean meats, poultry, egg yolks, sunflower seeds, pistachios, quail, pork), B2 (almonds, wild rice, venison, whole grains, molasses, egg yolks, legumes, nuts), B6 (brown rice, pinto beans, trout, sunflower seeds, whole grains, wheat germ, legumes, green leafy vegetables), B12 (fish, pork, eggs, milk), Choline (egg yolks, wheat germ, soybeans, fish, legumes), Folic Acid (dark green leafy vegetables, root vegetables, whole grains, oysters, salmon, milk), Niacin (peanuts, fish, lean meats, poultry, milk, rice bran), Pantothenic Acid (egg yolks, legumes, whole grains, wheat germ, salmon), C (raw fruits and vegetables), E (cold-pressed vegetable oils, egg, wheat germ, sweet potato, leaf vegetables), Calcium (milk, almonds, green leafy vegetables, shellfish), Magnesium (seafood, whole grains, dark green vegetables, nuts), Manganese (whole grains, green leafy vegetables, legumes, nuts, pineapple, egg yolk), Zinc (pumpkin seeds, sunflower seeds, seafood, mushrooms, soybeans, oysters, herring, eggs, wheat germ, lean meats)

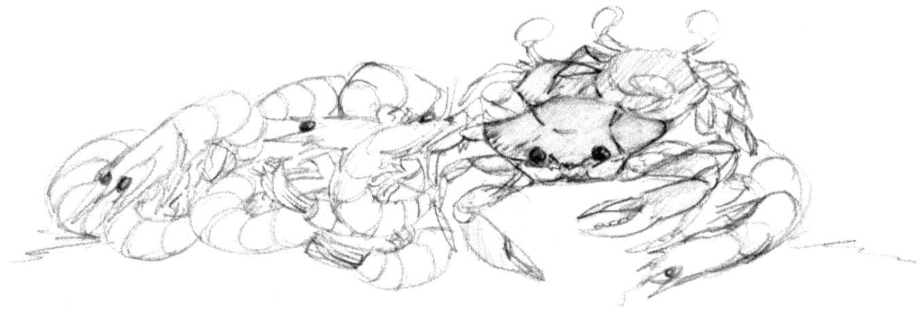

HYPERTENSION (HIGH BLOOD PRESSURE)

B group (including whole grains i.e. whole or ground wheat, whole or ground brown rice), Choline (egg yolks, wheat germ, soybeans, fish, legumes), Folic Acid (dark green leafy vegetables, root vegetables, whole grains, oysters, salmon, milk), Inositol (whole grains, citrus fruits, molasses, lean meats, milk, nuts, vegetables), Niacin (peanuts, milk, rice bran, lean meats, fish, poultry), Pangamic Acid (brown rice, sunflower seeds, pumpkin seeds, sesame seeds), Pantothenic Acid (egg yolks, legumes, whole grains, wheat germ, salmon) C (raw fruits and vegetables), D (salmon, sardines, herrings, egg yolks, organ meats), E (cold-pressed vegetable oils, egg, wheat germ, sweet potato, leaf vegetables), Bioflavonoids (citrus fruits, fruits, blackcurrants, buckwheat), Calcium (milk, almonds, green leafy vegetables, shellfish), Magnesium (seafood, whole grains, dark green vegetables, nuts), Potassium (lean meats, whole grains, vegetables, dried fruits, legumes, sunflower seeds, avocados, cantaloupes, plantains), Protein (lean meat, fish, poultry, soybeans, eggs, milk, whole grains), Fibre (bran)

HYPERTHYROIDISM

A (unprocessed orange vegetables and fruits), B group (including whole grains i.e. whole or ground wheat, whole or ground brown rice), Choline (egg yolks, wheat germ, soybeans, fish, legumes), Folic Acid (dark green leafy vegetables, root vegetables, whole grains, oysters, salmon, milk), Inositol (whole grains, citrus fruits, molasses, lean meats, milk, nuts, vegetables), C (raw fruits and vegetables), E (cold-pressed vegetable oils, egg, wheat germ, sweet potato, leaf vegetables), Calcium (milk, almonds, green leafy vegetables, shellfish), Iodine (seafood, kelp), Magnesium (seafood, whole grains, dark green vegetables, nuts), Carbohydrates (whole grains, fruits, vegetables), Protein (lean meat, fish, poultry, soybeans, eggs, milk, whole grains)

HYPOGLYCAEMIA (LOW BLOOD SUGAR)

A (unprocessed orange vegetables and fruits), B group (whole grains i.e. whole or ground wheat, whole or ground brown rice), B1 (whole grains, molasses, brown rice, fish, lean meats, poultry, egg yolks, sunflower seeds, pistachios, quail, pork), B2 (almonds, wild rice, venison, whole grains, molasses, egg yolks, legumes, nuts), B6 (brown rice, pinto beans, trout, sunflower seeds, whole grains, wheat germ, legumes, green leafy vegetables), B12 (fish, pork, eggs, milk), Biotin (egg yolks, unpolished rice, whole grains, sardines, legumes), Choline (egg yolks, wheat germ, soybeans, fish, legumes), Folic Acid (dark green leafy vegetables, root vegetables, whole grains, oysters, salmon, milk), Inositol (whole grains, citrus fruits, molasses, lean meats, milk, nuts, vegetables), Niacin (peanuts, fish, lean meats, poultry, milk, rice bran), PABA (wheat germ, plain, natural yogurt, molasses, green leafy vegetables), Pantothenic Acid (egg yolks, legumes, whole grains, wheat germ, salmon), C (raw fruits and vegetables), Bioflavonoids (citrus fruits, fruits, black currants, buckwheat), E (cold-pressed vegetable oils, egg, wheat germ, sweet potato, leaf vegetables), Calcium (milk, almonds, green leafy vegetables, shellfish), Chromium (grapes, raisins, corn oil, clams, whole grains), Copper (seafood, nuts, legumes, molasses, raisins), Iron (lean meats, fish, poultry, cherry juice, green leafy vegetables, dried fruits), Magnesium (seafood, whole grains, dark green vegetables, nuts), Manganese (whole grains, green leafy vegetables, legumes, nuts, pineapple, egg yolks, lima beans, sunflower seeds, tapioca, blackberries), Phosphorus (whole grains, fish, lean meats, poultry, eggs, milk, nuts), Potassium (lean meats, whole grains, vegetables, dried fruits, legumes, sunflower seeds, avocados, cantaloupes, plantains), Zinc (pumpkin seeds, sunflower seeds, seafood, mushrooms, soybeans, oysters, herring, eggs, wheat germ, lean meats), Methionine (quail, tuna, brazil nuts, goose, sesame seeds, lean meat), Protein (lean meat, fish, poultry, soybeans, eggs, milk, whole grains)

HYPOTENSION (LOW BLOOD PRESSURE)

A (unprocessed orange vegetables and fruits), B group (including whole grains i.e. whole or ground wheat, whole or ground brown rice), B1 (whole grains, molasses, brown rice, fish, lean meats, poultry, egg yolks, sunflower seeds, pistachios, quail, pork), Pantothenic Acid (egg yolks, legumes, whole grains, wheat germ, salmon), C (raw fruits and vegetables), D (salmon, sardines, herrings, egg yolks, organ meats), E (cold-pressed vegetable oils, egg, wheat germ, sweet potato, leaf vegetables), Manganese (whole grains, green leafy vegetables, legumes, nuts, pineapple, egg yolks, lima beans, sunflower seeds, tapioca, blackberries), Protein (lean meat, fish, poultry, soybeans, eggs, milk, whole grains)

HYPOTHYROIDISM

B group (including whole grains i.e. whole or ground wheat, whole or ground brown rice), B6 (lean meats, whole grains, molasses, wheat germ, legumes, green leafy vegetables), Choline (egg yolks, wheat germ, soybeans, fish, legumes), C (raw fruits and vegetables), E (cold-pressed vegetable oils, egg, wheat germ, sweet potato, leaf vegetables), Iodine (seafood or 1 teaspoon kelp), Protein (lean meat, fish, poultry, soybeans, eggs, milk, whole grains)

INDIGESTION (DYSPEPSIA)

B group (including whole grains i.e. whole or ground wheat, whole or ground brown rice), B1 (whole grains, molasses, brown rice, fish, lean meats, poultry, egg yolks, sunflower seeds, pistachios, quail, pork), B6 (brown rice, pinto beans, trout, sunflower seeds, whole grains, wheat germ, legumes, green leafy vegetables), Folic Acid (dark green leafy vegetables, root vegetables, whole grains, oysters, salmon, milk), Niacin (peanuts, fish, lean meats, poultry, milk, rice bran), Pantothenic Acid (egg yolks, legumes, whole grains, wheat germ, salmon), plain natural yogurt

INFECTIONS

A (unprocessed orange vegetables and fruits), B group (including whole grains i.e. whole or ground wheat, whole or ground brown rice), B6 (brown rice, pinto beans, trout, sunflower seeds, whole grains, wheat germ, legumes, green leafy vegetables, Pantothenic Acid (egg yolks, legumes, whole grains, wheat germ, salmon), C (raw fruits and vegetables), Protein (lean meat, fish, poultry, soybeans, eggs, milk, whole grains), plain natural yogurt

INSOMNIA (SLEEPLESSNESS)

B group (whole grains i.e. whole or ground wheat, whole or ground brown rice), B6 (brown rice, pinto beans, trout, sunflower seeds, whole grains, wheat germ, legumes, green leafy vegetables), B12 (fish, pork, eggs, milk), Inositol (whole grains, citrus fruits, molasses, lean meats, milk, nuts, vegetables), Niacin (peanuts, fish, lean meats, poultry, milk, rice bran), Pantothenic Acid (egg yolks, legumes, whole grains, wheat germ, salmon), C (raw fruits and vegetables), D (salmon, sardines, herrings, egg yolks, organ meats), E (cold-pressed vegetable oils, egg, wheat germ, sweet potato, leaf vegetables), Calcium (milk, almonds, green leafy vegetables, shellfish), Magnesium (seafood, whole grains, dark green vegetables, nuts), Phosphorus (whole grains, fish, lean meats, poultry, eggs, milk, nuts), Potassium (lean meats, whole grains, vegetables, dried fruits, legumes, sunflower seeds, avocados, cantaloupes, plantains), Tryptophan (bananas, milk)

INTESTINAL PARASITES

A (unprocessed orange vegetables and fruits), B1 (whole grains, molasses, brown rice, fish, lean meats, poultry, egg yolks, sunflower seeds, pistachios, quail, pork), B2 (almonds, wild rice, venison, whole grains, molasses, egg yolks, legumes, nuts), B group (whole grains i.e. whole or ground wheat, whole or ground brown rice), B6 (brown rice, pinto beans, trout, sunflower seeds, whole grains, wheat germ, legumes, green leafy vegetables), B12 (fish, pork, eggs, milk), Pantothenic Acid (egg yolks, legumes, whole grains, wheat germ, salmon), C (raw fruits and vegetables), D (salmon, sardines, herrings, egg yolks, organ meats), K (green leafy vegetables, egg yolks, safflower oil, molasses, cauliflower, soybeans), Calcium (milk, almonds, green leafy vegetables, shellfish), Iron (lean meats, fish, poultry, cherry juice, green leafy vegetables, dried fruits), Potassium (lean meats, whole grains, vegetables, dried fruits, legumes, sunflower seeds, avocados, cantaloupes, plantains), Sulfur (fish, red hot peppers, garlic, onions, eggs, lean meats, cabbage, brussel sprouts, horseradish), Protein (lean meat, fish, poultry, soybeans, eggs, milk, whole grains), Unsaturated fatty acids (vegetable oils, sunflower seeds), plain natural yogurt

JAUNDICE

A (unprocessed orange vegetables and fruits), B Group (including whole grains i.e. whole or ground wheat, whole or ground brown rice), B6 (brown rice, pinto beans, trout, sunflower seeds, whole grains, wheat germ, legumes, green leafy vegetables), C (raw fruits and vegetables), D (salmon, sardines, herrings, egg yolks, organ meats), E (cold-pressed vegetable oils, egg, wheat germ, sweet potato, leaf vegetables), Choline (egg yolks, wheat germ, soybeans, fish, legumes), Folic Acid (dark green leafy vegetables, root vegetables, whole grains, oysters, salmon, milk), Niacin (peanuts, fish, lean meats, poultry, milk, rice bran), Pantothenic Acid (egg yolks, legumes, whole grains, wheat germ, salmon), Calcium (milk, almonds, green leafy vegetables, shellfish), Magnesium (seafood, whole grains, dark green vegetables, nuts), Phosphorus (fish, lean meats, poultry, eggs, milk, nuts, whole grains), Protein (lean meat, fish, poultry, soybeans, eggs, milk, whole grains), Unsaturated fatty acids (vegetable oils, sunflower seeds)

KIDNEY DISEASES

A (unprocessed orange vegetables and fruits), B group (including whole grains i.e. whole or ground wheat, whole or ground brown rice), C (raw fruits and vegetables), Bioflavonoids (citrus fruits, fruits, blackcurrants, buckwheat), E (cold-pressed vegetable oils, egg, wheat germ, sweet potato, leaf vegetables), Potassium (lean meats, whole grains, vegetables, dried fruits, legumes, sunflower seeds, avocados, cantaloupes or rockmelons, plantains)

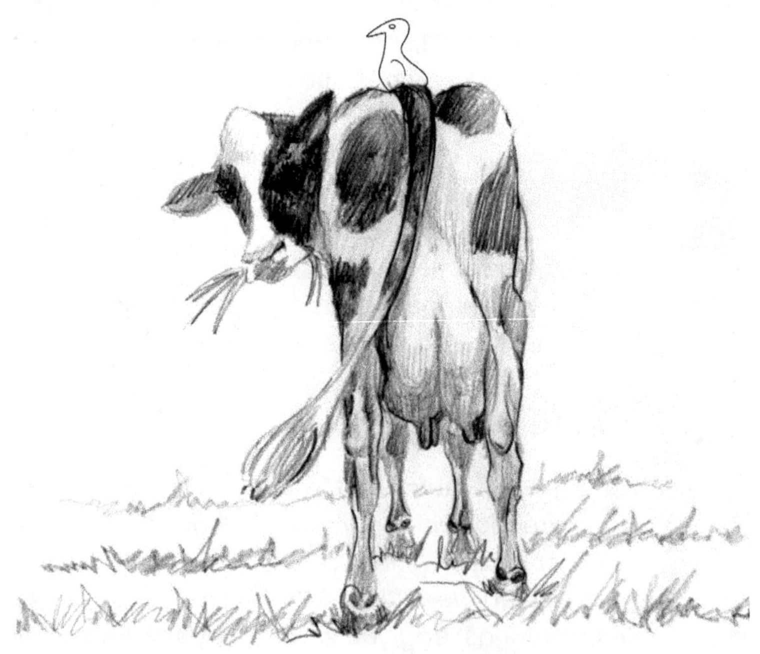

KIDNEY STONES (RENAL CALCULI)

A (unprocessed orange vegetables and fruits), B2 (almonds, wild rice, venison, whole grains, molasses, egg yolks, legumes, nuts), B6 (brown rice, pinto beans, trout, sunflower seeds, whole grains, wheat germ, legumes, green leafy vegetables), C (raw fruits and vegetables), E (cold-pressed vegetable oils, egg, wheat germ, sweet potato, leaf vegetables), Magnesium (seafood, whole grains, dark green vegetables, nuts), Decrease fats

KWASHIORKOR

A (unprocessed orange vegetables and fruits), Folic Acid (dark-green vegetables, root vegetables, whole grains, oysters, salmon, milk), C (raw fruits and vegetables), D (salmon, sardines, herrings, egg yolks, organ meats), E (cold-pressed vegetable oils, egg, wheat germ, sweet potato, leaf vegetables), Chromium (grapes, raisins, corn oil, clams, whole grains), Copper (seafood, nuts, legumes, molasses, raisins), Iron (lean meats, fish, poultry, cherry juice, green leafy vegetables, dried fruits), Magnesium (seafood, whole grains, dark green vegetables, nuts), Selenium (tuna, herring, wheat germ, wheat bran, whole grains, sesame seeds), Protein (lean meat, fish, poultry, soybeans, eggs, milk, whole grains)

LEG CRAMP

B group (whole grains i.e. whole or ground wheat, whole or ground brown rice), B1 (whole grains, molasses, brown rice, fish, lean meats, poultry, egg yolks, sunflower seeds, pistachios, quail, pork), B2 (almonds, wild rice, venison, whole grains, molasses, egg yolks, legumes, nuts), Biotin (egg yolks, unpolished rice, whole grains, sardines, legumes), Pantothenic Acid (egg yolks, legumes, whole grains, wheat germ, salmon), C (raw fruits and vegetables), D (salmon, sardines, herrings, egg yolks, organ meats), E (cold-pressed vegetable oils, egg, wheat germ, sweet potato, leaf vegetables), Calcium (milk, almonds, green leafy vegetables, shellfish), Magnesium (seafood, whole grains, dark-green vegetables, nuts), Phosphorus (fish, lean meats, poultry, eggs, milk, nuts, whole grains), Sodium (seafood, celery, kelp), Protein (lean meat, fish, poultry, soybeans, eggs, milk, whole grains), Unsaturated fatty acids (vegetable oils, sunflower seeds)

LEUKAEMIA

B group (whole grains i.e. whole or ground wheat, whole or ground brown rice), B12 (fish, pork, eggs, milk), Folic Acid (dark green leafy vegetables, root vegetables, whole grains, oysters, salmon, milk), C (raw fruits and vegetables), E (cold-pressed vegetable oils, egg, wheat germ, sweet potato, leaf vegetables), Bioflavonoids (citrus fruits, fruits, blackcurrants, buckwheat), Copper (seafood, nuts, legumes, molasses, raisins), Iron (lean meats, eggs, fish, poultry, molasses, cherry juice, green leafy vegetables), Zinc (pumpkin seeds, sunflower seeds, seafood, mushrooms, soybeans, oysters, herring, eggs, wheat germ, lean meats)

Please note: If someone consistently experiences exposure to high electromagnetic fields' (EMFs) that person could be at risk in developing health problems including leukaemia and cancer (NCRP Scientific Committee, 1995). The Swedish Government has established a safety limit at 2.5mG and this standard is accepted throughout the world. Currently, there are no legally enforceable Australian standards regulating environmental exposures. Because EMFs cannot be seen, the only way to determine if they are a problem is with relevant equipment and training (Bijlsma, 2010). It is important to minimise EMFs where you sleep and where you spend long periods of time sitting. According to Lucinda Grant (1997), a recent Electrical Sensitivity (ES) survey revealed the five most common symptoms experienced when EMF exposed were skin itch/rash/flushing/burning and/or tingling, confusion/poor concentration and/or memory loss, fatigue/weakness, headache, and chest pain/heart problems. Less common were nausea, panic attacks, insomnia, seizures, ear pain/ringing in the ears, feeling a vibration, paralysis, and dizziness.

LIVER DISORDERS

A (unprocessed orange vegetables and fruits), B group (whole grains i.e. whole or ground wheat, whole or ground brown rice), B1 (whole grains, molasses, brown rice, fish, lean meats, poultry, egg yolks, sunflower seeds, pistachios, quail, pork), B2 (almonds, wild rice, venison, whole grains, molasses, egg yolks, legumes, nuts), B6 (brown rice, pinto beans, trout, sunflower seeds, whole grains, wheat germ, legumes, green leafy vegetables), Choline (egg yolks, wheat germ, soybeans, fish, legumes),

Niacin (peanuts, fish, lean meats, poultry, milk, rice bran), Pantothenic Acid (egg yolks, legumes, whole grains, wheat germ, salmon), C (raw fruits and vegetables), E (cold-pressed vegetable oils, egg, wheat germ, sweet potato, leaf vegetables), Calcium (milk, almonds, green leafy vegetables, shellfish), Magnesium (seafood, whole grains, dark green vegetables, nuts), Protein (lean meat, fish, poultry, soybeans, eggs, milk, whole grains), plain natural yogurt

LUNGS/RESPIRATORY SYSTEM:

B1 (whole grains, brown rice, lean meats, fish, poultry, egg yolks), C (raw fruits and vegetables), E (cold-pressed vegetable oils, eggs, wheat germ, sweet potato, leafy vegetables), Calcium (skim milk, green leafy vegetables, shellfish), Magnesium (seafood, whole grains, dark green vegetables, molasses, nuts), Selenium (tuna, herring, wheat germ, wheat bran, whole grains, sesame seeds)

MEASLES

A (unprocessed orange vegetables and fruits), C (raw fruits and vegetables), E (cold-pressed vegetable oils, egg, wheat germ, sweet potato, leaf vegetables, cucumber), Protein (lean meat, fish, poultry, soybeans, eggs, milk, whole grains)

MÈNIÈRE'S SYNDROME

B group (whole grains i.e. whole or ground wheat, whole or ground brown rice), B1 (whole grains, molasses, brown rice, fish, lean meats, poultry, egg yolks, sunflower seeds, pistachios, quail, pork), B6 (brown rice, pinto beans, trout, sunflower seeds, whole grains, wheat germ, legumes, green leafy vegetables), Niacin (peanuts, fish, lean meats, poultry, milk, rice bran), E (cold-pressed vegetable oils, egg, wheat germ, sweet potato, leaf vegetables), Calcium (milk, almonds, green leafy vegetables, shellfish), Unsaturated fatty acids (vegetable oils, sunflower seeds)

MENINGITIS

A (unprocessed orange vegetables and fruits), C (raw fruits and vegetables), D (salmon, sardines, herrings, egg yolks, organ meats), Calcium (milk, almonds, green leafy vegetables, shellfish), Protein (lean meat, fish, poultry, soybeans, eggs, milk, whole grains)

MONONUCLEOSIS

A (unprocessed orange vegetables and fruits), B group (whole grains i.e. whole or ground wheat, whole or ground brown rice), B1 (whole grains, molasses, brown rice, fish, lean meats, poultry, egg yolks, sunflower seeds, pistachios, quail, pork), B2 (almonds, wild rice, venison, whole grains, molasses, egg yolks, legumes, nuts), B6 (brown rice, pinto beans, trout, sunflower seeds, whole grains, wheat germ, legumes, green leafy vegetables), Biotin (egg yolks, unpolished rice, whole grains, sardines, legumes), Choline (egg yolks, wheat germ, soybeans, fish, legumes), Pantothenic Acid (egg yolks, legumes, whole grains, wheat germ, salmon), C (raw fruits and vegetables), Potassium (lean meats, whole grains, vegetables, dried fruits, legumes, sunflower seeds, avocados, cantaloupes, plantains), Protein (lean meat, fish, poultry, soybeans, eggs, milk, whole grains)

MOUTH AND TONGUE DISORDERS

B group (whole grains i.e. whole or ground wheat, whole or ground brown rice), C (raw fruits and vegetables), plain natural yogurt

MULTIPLE SCLEROSIS

B group (whole grains i.e. whole or ground wheat, whole or ground brown rice), B1 (whole grains, molasses, brown rice, fish, lean meats, poultry, egg yolks, sunflower seeds, pistachios, quail, pork), B2 (almonds, wild rice, venison, whole grains, molasses, egg yolks, legumes, nuts), B6 (brown rice, pinto beans, trout, sunflower seeds, whole grains, wheat germ, legumes, green leafy vegetables), B12 (fish, pork, eggs, milk), Choline (egg yolks, wheat germ, soybeans, fish, legumes), Niacin (peanuts, fish, lean meats, poultry, milk, rice bran), Pangamic Acid (brown rice, sunflower seeds, pumpkin seeds, sesame seeds), Pantothenic Acid (egg yolks, legumes, whole grains, wheat germ, salmon), C (raw fruits and vegetables), E (cold-pressed vegetable oils, egg, wheat germ, sweet potato, leaf vegetables), Calcium (milk, almonds, green leafy vegetables, shellfish), Copper (seafood, nuts, legumes, molasses, raisins), Iron (lean meats, fish, poultry, cherry juice, green leafy vegetables, dried fruits), Magnesium (seafood, whole grains, dark green vegetables, nuts), Manganese (whole grains, green leafy vegetables, legumes, nuts, pineapple, egg yolks, lima beans, sunflower seeds, tapioca, blackberries), Selenium (tuna, herring, wheat germ, wheat bran, whole grains, sesame seeds), Zinc (pumpkin seeds, sunflower seeds, seafood, mushrooms, soybeans, oysters, herring, eggs, wheat germ, lean meats), Protein (lean meat, fish, poultry, soybeans, eggs, milk, whole grains), Unsaturated fatty acids 2 tablespoons (vegetable oils, sunflower seeds)

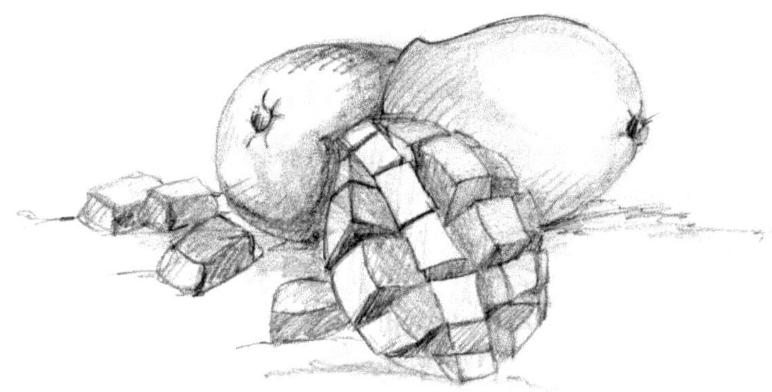

MUSCLE WEAKNESS

E (cold-pressed vegetable oils, egg, wheat germ, sweet potato, leaf vegetables, cucumber), Manganese (whole grains, green leafy vegetables, legumes, nuts, pineapple, egg yolks), Potassium (lean meats, whole grains, vegetables, dried fruits, legumes, sunflower seeds, avocados, cantaloupes, plantains), Zinc (pumpkin seeds, sunflower seeds, seafood, mushrooms, soybeans, oysters, herring, eggs, wheat germ, lean meats), Unsaturated fatty acids (vegetable oils, sunflower seeds), Protein (lean meat, fish, poultry, soybeans, eggs, milk, whole grains)

MUSCULAR DYSTROPHY

A (unprocessed orange vegetables and fruits), B group (whole grains i.e. whole or ground wheat, whole or ground brown rice), B6 (brown rice, pinto beans, trout, sunflower seeds, whole grains, wheat germ, legumes, green leafy vegetables), B12 (fish, pork, eggs, milk), Choline (egg yolks, wheat germ, soybeans, fish, legumes), Niacin (peanuts, fish, lean meats, poultry, milk, rice bran), Pantothenic Acid (egg yolks, legumes, whole grains, wheat germ, salmon), C (raw fruits and vegetables), E (cold-pressed vegetable oils, egg, wheat germ, sweet potato, leaf vegetables), Potassium (lean meats, whole grains, vegetables, dried fruits, legumes, sunflower seeds, avocados, cantaloupes, plantains), Protein (lean meat, fish, poultry, soybeans, eggs, milk, whole grains), Unsaturated fatty acids (vegetable oils, sunflower seeds)

MYASTHENIA GRAVIS

B group (whole grains i.e. whole or ground wheat, whole or ground brown rice), B1 (whole grains, molasses, brown rice, fish, lean meats, poultry, egg yolks, sunflower seeds, pistachios, quail, pork), B2 (almonds, wild rice, venison, whole grains, molasses, egg yolks, legumes, nuts), B6 (brown rice, pinto beans, trout, sunflower seeds, whole grains, wheat germ, legumes, green leafy vegetables), B12 (fish, pork, eggs, milk), Choline (egg yolks, wheat germ, soybeans, fish, legumes), Folic Acid (dark green leafy vegetables, root vegetables, whole grains, oysters, salmon, milk), Inositol (whole grains, citrus fruits, molasses, lean meats, milk, nuts, vegetables), Pantothenic Acid (egg yolks, legumes, whole grains, wheat germ, salmon), C (raw fruits and vegetables), E (cold-pressed vegetable oils, egg, wheat germ, sweet potato, leaf vegetables), Magnesium (seafood, whole grains, dark green vegetables, nuts), Manganese (whole grains, green leafy vegetables, legumes, nuts, pineapple, egg yolks, lima beans, sunflower seeds, tapioca, blackberries), Potassium (lean meats, whole grains, vegetables, dried fruits, legumes, sunflower seeds, avocados, cantaloupes, plantains), Sodium - for a short period (kelp), Protein (lean meat, fish, poultry, soybeans, eggs, milk, whole grains); Please note: Breakfast needs to be the most nutritionally dense meal of the day consisting of soft-textured foods. Small and frequent meals during the day may need a half hour rest period before each serving.

NAIL PROBLEMS

A (unprocessed orange vegetables and fruits), B group (whole grains i.e. whole or ground wheat, whole or ground brown rice), Folic Acid (dark green leafy vegetables, root vegetables, whole grains, oysters, salmon, milk), C (raw fruits and vegetables), Calcium (milk, almonds, green leafy vegetables, shellfish), Iron (lean meats, fish, poultry, cherry juice, green leafy vegetables, dried fruits), Zinc (pumpkin seeds, sunflower seeds, seafood, mushrooms, soybeans, oysters, herring, eggs, wheat germ, lean meats), Protein (lean meat, fish, poultry, soybean, eggs, milk, whole grains)

NAUSEA AND VOMITING

B group (whole grains i.e. whole or ground wheat, whole or ground brown rice), B6 (brown rice, pinto beans, trout, sunflower seeds, whole grains, wheat germ, legumes, green leafy vegetables), Magnesium (seafood, whole grains, dark green vegetables, nuts)

NEPHRITIS (KIDNEY INFECTION)

A (unprocessed orange vegetables and fruits), B group (whole grains i.e. whole or ground wheat, whole or ground brown rice), B2 (almonds, wild rice, venison, whole grains, molasses, egg yolks, legumes, nuts), B12 (fish, pork, eggs, milk), Choline (egg yolks, wheat germ, soybeans, fish, legumes), Niacin (peanuts, fish, lean meats, poultry, milk, rice bran), Folic Acid (dark green leafy vegetables, root vegetables, whole grains, oysters, salmon, milk), Inositol (whole grains, citrus fruits, molasses, lean meats, milk, nuts, vegetables), Pantothenic Acid (egg yolks, legumes, whole grains, wheat germ, salmon), C (raw fruits and vegetables), E (cold-pressed vegetable oils, egg, wheat germ, sweet potato, leaf vegetables), Calcium (milk, almonds, green leafy vegetables, shellfish), Iron (lean meats, fish, poultry, cherry juice, green leafy vegetables, dried fruits), Magnesium (seafood, whole grains, dark green vegetables, nuts), Fluids (filtered rain water, herbal teas), Protein (lean meat, fish, poultry, soybeans, eggs, milk, whole grains)

NEURITIS

B group (whole grains i.e. whole or ground wheat, whole or ground brown rice), B1 (whole grains, molasses, brown rice, fish, lean meats, poultry, egg yolks, sunflower seeds, pistachios, quail, pork), B2 (almonds, wild rice, venison, whole grains, molasses, egg yolks, legumes, nuts), B6 (brown rice, pinto beans, trout, sunflower seeds, whole grains, wheat germ, legumes, green leafy vegetables), B12 (fish, pork, eggs, milk), Niacin (peanuts, fish, lean meats, poultry, milk, rice bran), Pantothenic Acid (egg yolks, legumes, whole grains, wheat germ, salmon), Calcium (milk, almonds, green leafy vegetables, shellfish), Magnesium (seafood, whole grains, dark green vegetables, nuts), Protein (lean meat, fish, poultry, soybeans, eggs, milk, whole grains)

OSTEOPOROSIS (BRITTLE BONES)

B12 (fish, pork, eggs, milk), C (raw fruits and vegetables), D (salmon, sardines, herrings, egg yolks, organ meats), E (cold-pressed vegetable oils, egg, wheat germ, sweet potato, leaf vegetables), Calcium (milk, almonds, green leafy vegetables, shellfish), Copper (seafood, nuts, legumes, raisins), Fluoride (tea, seafood), Magnesium (seafood, whole grains, dark-green vegetables, nuts), Phosphorus (fish, lean meats, poultry, eggs, milk, nuts, whole grains), Protein (lean meat, fish, poultry, soybeans, eggs, milk, whole grains)

OVERWEIGHT AND OBESITY

B group (whole grains i.e. whole or ground wheat, whole or ground brown rice), B2 (almonds, wild rice, venison, whole grains, molasses, egg yolks, legumes, nuts), B6 (brown rice, pinto beans, trout, sunflower seeds, whole grains, wheat germ, legumes, green leafy vegetables), B12 (fish, pork, eggs, milk), Choline (egg yolks, wheat germ, soybeans, fish, legumes), Folic Acid (dark green leafy vegetables, root vegetables, whole grains, oysters, salmon, milk), Inositol (whole grains, citrus fruits, molasses, lean meats, milk, nuts, vegetables), Pantothenic Acid (egg yolks, legumes, whole grains, wheat germ, salmon), C (raw fruits and vegetables), E (cold-pressed vegetable oils, egg, wheat germ, sweet potato, leaf vegetables), Calcium (milk, almonds, green leafy vegetables, shellfish), Magnesium (seafood, whole grains, dark green vegetables, nuts), Phosphorus (fish, lean meats, poultry, eggs, milk, nuts, whole grains), Protein (lean meat, fish, poultry, soybeans, eggs, milk, whole grains), Unsaturated fatty acids (vegetable oils, sunflower seeds)

PANCREATITIS

B group (whole grains i.e. whole or ground wheat, whole or ground brown rice), B6 (brown rice, pinto beans, trout, sunflower seeds, whole grains, wheat germ, legumes, green leafy vegetables), E (cold-pressed vegetable oils, egg, wheat germ, sweet potato, leaf vegetables), plain natural yogurt

PARKINSON'S DISEASE

B group (whole grains i.e. whole or ground wheat, whole or ground brown rice), B2 (almonds, wild rice, venison, whole grains, molasses, egg yolks, legumes, nuts), B6 (brown rice, pinto beans, trout, sunflower seeds, whole grains, wheat germ, legumes, green leafy vegetables), Niacin (peanuts, fish, lean meats, poultry, milk, rice bran), C (raw fruits and vegetables), E (cold-pressed vegetable oils, egg, wheat germ, sweet potato, leaf vegetables), Calcium (milk, almonds, green leafy vegetables, shellfish), Magnesium (seafood, whole grains, dark green vegetables, nuts), Protein (lean meat, fish, poultry, soybeans, eggs, milk, whole grains)

PELLAGRA

Niacin (peanuts, fish, lean meats, poultry, milk, rice bran), B group (whole grains i.e. whole or ground wheat, whole or ground brown rice), B1 (whole grains, molasses, brown rice, fish, lean meats, poultry, egg yolks, sunflower seeds, pistachios, quail, pork), B2 (almonds, wild rice, venison, whole grains, molasses, egg yolks, legumes, nuts), B12 (fish, pork, eggs, milk), Folic Acid (dark-green leafy vegetables, root vegetables, whole grains, oysters, salmon, milk), Protein (lean meat, fish, poultry, soybeans, eggs, milk, whole grains), Tryptophan (bananas, milk)

PERIODONTAL DISEASE

C (raw fruits and vegetables), Folic Acid (dark green leafy vegetables, root vegetables, whole grains, oysters, salmon, milk), Zinc (pumpkin seeds, sunflower seeds, seafood, mushrooms, soybeans, oysters, herring, eggs, wheat germ, lean meats), Protein (lean meat, fish, poultry, soybeans, eggs, milk, whole grains), A (unprocessed orange vegetables and fruits); Good oral hygiene habits reduce risk of decay.

PERNICIOUS ANAEMIA

B group (including whole grains i.e. whole or ground wheat, whole or ground brown rice), B6 (brown rice, pinto beans, trout, sunflower seeds, whole grains, wheat germ, legumes, green leafy vegetables), B12 (fish, pork, eggs, milk), Folic Acid (dark green leafy vegetables, root vegetables, whole grains, oysters, salmon, milk), C (raw fruits and vegetables), E (cold-pressed vegetable oils, egg, wheat germ, sweet potato, leaf vegetables), Calcium (milk, almonds, green leafy vegetables, shellfish),

Cobalt (oysters, clams, poultry, milk, green leafy vegetables, fruits), Protein (lean meat, fish, poultry, soybeans, eggs, milk, whole grains)

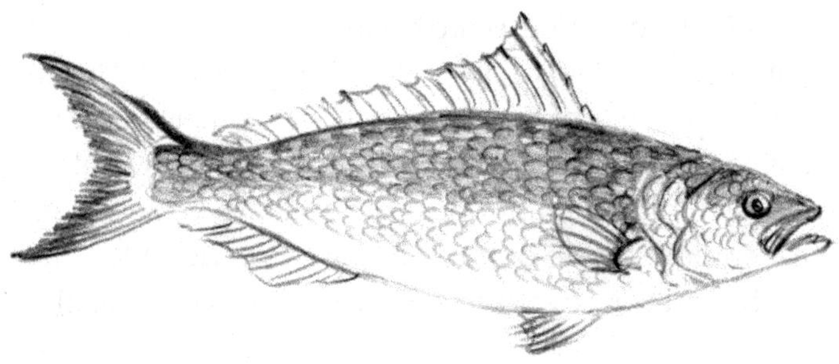

PHLEBITIS

B group (whole grains i.e. whole or ground wheat, whole or ground brown rice), Niacin (peanuts, fish, lean meats, poultry, milk, rice bran), Pantothenic Acid (egg yolks, legumes, whole grains, wheat germ, salmon), C (raw fruits and vegetables), E (cold-pressed vegetable oils, egg, wheat germ, sweet potato, leaf vegetables), Calcium (milk, almonds, green leafy vegetables, shellfish)

PNEUMONIA

A (unprocessed orange vegetables and fruits), B group (whole grains i.e. whole or ground wheat, whole or ground brown rice), C (raw fruits and vegetables), D (salmon, sardines, herrings, egg yolks, organ meats), E (cold-pressed vegetable oils, egg, wheat germ, sweet potato, leaf vegetables), K (green leafy vegetables, egg yolks, safflower oil, molasses, cauliflower, soybeans), Bioflavonoids (citrus fruits, fruits, blackcurrants, buckwheat), Protein (lean meat, fish, poultry, soybeans, eggs, milk, whole grains), Calcium (milk, almonds, green leafy vegetables, shellfish)

POLIO

A (unprocessed orange vegetables and fruits), B group (whole grains i.e. whole or ground wheat, whole or ground brown rice), C (raw fruits and vegetables), Calcium (milk, almonds, green leafy vegetables, shellfish), Magnesium (seafood, whole grains, dark green vegetables, nuts), Potassium (lean meats, whole grains, vegetables, dried fruits, legumes, sunflower seeds, avocados, cantaloupes, plantains), Sodium (seafood, celery, kelp), Protein (lean meat, fish, poultry, soybeans, eggs, milk, whole grains)

PROSTATITIS

A (unprocessed orange vegetables and fruits), B group (whole grains i.e. whole or ground wheat, whole or ground brown rice), B6 (brown rice, pinto beans, trout, sunflower seeds, whole grains, wheat germ, legumes, green leafy vegetables), C (raw fruits and vegetables), E (cold-pressed vegetable oils, egg, wheat germ, sweet potato, leaf vegetables), Magnesium (seafood, whole grains, dark-green vegetables, nuts), Zinc (pumpkin seeds, sunflower seeds, seafood, mushrooms, soybeans, oysters, herring, eggs, wheat germ, lean meats), Unsaturated fatty acids (vegetable oils, sunflower seeds), Protein (lean meat, fish, poultry, soybeans, eggs, milk, whole grains), filtered, detoxified rainwater

PRURITIS ANI

A (unprocessed orange vegetables and fruits), B group (whole grains i.e. whole or ground wheat, whole or ground brown rice), Iron (lean meats, fish, poultry, cherry juice, green leafy vegetables, dried fruits), plain natural yogurt

PSORIASIS

A (unprocessed orange vegetables and fruits), B group (whole grains i.e. whole or ground wheat, whole or ground brown rice), B2 (almonds, wild rice, venison, whole grains, molasses, egg yolks, legumes, nuts), B6 (brown rice, pinto beans, trout, sunflower seeds, whole grains, wheat germ, legumes, green leafy vegetables, B12 (fish, pork, eggs, milk), Folic Acid (dark-green leafy vegetables, root vegetables, whole grains, oysters, salmon, milk), Pantothenic Acid (egg yolks, legumes, whole grains, wheat germ, salmon), C (raw fruits and vegetables), D (salmon, sardines, herrings, egg yolks, organ meats), E (cold-pressed vegetable oils, egg, wheat germ, sweet potato, leaf vegetables), Bioflavonoids (citrus fruits, fruits, blackcurrants, buckwheat), Magnesium (seafood, whole grains, dark green vegetables, nuts), Sulphur (fish, red hot peppers, garlic, onions, eggs, lean meats, cabbage, brussel sprouts, horseradish) Zinc (pumpkin seeds, sunflower seeds, seafood, mushrooms, soybeans, oysters, herring, eggs, wheat germ, lean meats), Unsaturated fatty acids (vegetable oils, sunflower seeds)

PYELONEPHRITIS

Cranberries, blueberries; Substances seem to inhibit the adherence of *Escherichia coli* bacteria to the epithelial cells of the urinary tract (Mahan & Escott-Stump, 1996)

PYORRHEA (SORE GUMS)

A (unprocessed orange vegetables and fruits), B group (whole grains i.e. whole or ground wheat, whole or ground brown rice), B1 (whole grains, molasses, brown rice, fish, lean meats, poultry, egg yolks, sunflower seeds, pistachios, quail, pork), B2 (almonds, wild rice, venison, whole grains, molasses, egg yolks, legumes, nuts), B6 (brown rice, pinto beans, trout, sunflower seeds, whole grains, wheat germ, legumes, green leafy vegetables), Biotin (egg yolks, unpolished rice, whole grains, sardines, legumes), Folic Acid (dark-green leafy vegetables, root vegetables, whole grains, oysters, salmon, milk), Niacin (peanuts, fish, lean meats, poultry, milk, rice bran), Pantothenic Acid (egg yolks, legumes, whole grains, wheat germ, salmon), C (raw fruits and vegetables), D (salmon, sardines, herrings, egg yolks, organ meats), Bioflavonoids (citrus fruits, fruits, blackcurrants, buckwheat), Calcium (milk, almonds, green leafy vegetables, shellfish), Magnesium (seafood, whole grains, dark green vegetables, nuts), Manganese (whole grains, green leafy vegetables, legumes, nuts, pineapple, egg yolks, lima beans, sunflower seeds, tapioca, blackberries), Zinc (pumpkin seeds, sunflower seeds, seafood, mushrooms, soybeans, oysters, herring, eggs, wheat germ, lean meats), Protein (lean meat, fish, poultry, soybeans, eggs, milk, whole grains)

RHEUMATIC FEVER

A (unprocessed orange vegetables and fruits), B group (whole grains i.e. whole or ground wheat, whole or ground brown rice), B2 (almonds, wild rice, venison, whole grains, molasses, egg yolks, legumes, nuts), B6 (brown rice, pinto beans, trout, sunflower seeds, whole grains, wheat germ, legumes, green leafy vegetables), Pantothenic Acid (egg yolks, legumes, whole grains, wheat germ, salmon), Pangamic Acid, C (raw fruits and vegetables), D (salmon, sardines, herrings, egg yolks, organ meats),

E (cold-pressed vegetable oils, egg, wheat germ, sweet potato, leaf vegetables), Bioflavonoids (citrus fruits, fruits, blackcurrants, buckwheat), Zinc (pumpkin seeds, sunflower seeds, seafood, mushrooms, soybeans, oysters, herring, eggs, wheat germ, lean meats), Protein (lean meat, fish, poultry, soybeans, eggs, milk, whole grains)

RHEUMATISM

A (unprocessed orange vegetables and fruits), B group (whole grains i.e. whole or ground wheat, whole or ground brown rice), B6 (brown rice, pinto beans, trout, sunflower seeds, whole grains, wheat germ, legumes, green leafy vegetables), Pangamic Acid (brown rice, sunflower seeds, pumpkin seeds, sesame seeds), Pantothenic Acid (egg yolks, legumes, whole grains, wheat germ, salmon), C (raw fruits and vegetables), D (salmon, sardines, herrings, egg yolks, organ meats), E (cold-pressed vegetable oils, egg, wheat germ, sweet potato, leaf vegetables), Bioflavonoids (citrus fruits, fruits, blackcurrants, buckwheat), Calcium (milk, almonds, green leafy vegetables, shellfish), Phosphorus (fish, lean meats, poultry, eggs, milk, nuts, whole grains), Potassium (lean meats, whole grains, vegetables, dried fruits, legumes, sunflower seeds, avocados, cantaloupes, plantains), Zinc (pumpkin seeds, sunflower seeds, seafood, mushrooms, soybeans, oysters, herring, eggs, wheat germ, lean meats), Protein (lean meat, fish, poultry, soybeans, eggs, milk, whole grains)

RICKETS AND OSTEOMALACIA

A (unprocessed orange vegetables and fruits), C (raw fruits and vegetables), D (salmon, sardines, herrings, egg yolks, organ meats), Calcium (milk, almonds, green leafy vegetables, shellfish), Magnesium (seafood, whole grains, dark green vegetables, nuts), Phosphorus (fish, lean meats, poultry, eggs, milk, nuts, whole grains), Unsaturated fatty acids (vegetable oils, sunflower seeds)

RHINITIS

A (unprocessed orange vegetables and fruits), C (raw fruits and vegetables), Protein (lean meat, fish, poultry, soybeans, eggs, milk, whole grains)

SCIATICA

B Group (whole grains i.e. whole or ground wheat, whole or ground brown rice), B1 (whole grains, molasses, brown rice, fish, lean meats, poultry, egg yolks, sunflower seeds, pistachios, quail, pork), B12 (fish, pork, eggs, milk), D (salmon, sardines, herrings, egg yolks, organ meats), E (cold-pressed vegetable oils, egg, wheat germ, sweet potato, leaf vegetables)

SCURVY

A (unprocessed orange vegetables and fruits), B group (whole grains i.e. whole or ground wheat, whole or ground brown rice), Folic Acid (dark green leafy vegetables, root vegetables, whole grains, oysters, salmon, milk), C (raw fruits and vegetables), D (salmon, sardines, herrings, egg yolks, organ meats), Bioflavonoids (citrus fruits, fruits, blackcurrants, buckwheat), Calcium (milk, almonds, green leafy vegetables, shellfish), Iron (lean meats, fish, poultry, cherry juice, green leafy vegetables, dried fruits), Magnesium (seafood, whole grains, dark green vegetables, nuts), Protein (lean meat, fish, poultry, soybeans, eggs, milk, whole grains)

SHINGLES (HERPES ZOSTER)

A (unprocessed orange vegetables and fruits), B group (whole grains i.e. whole or ground wheat, whole or ground brown rice), B1 (whole grains, molasses, brown rice, fish, lean meats, poultry, egg yolks, sunflower seeds, pistachios, quail, pork), B6 (brown rice, pinto beans, trout, sunflower seeds, whole grains, wheat germ, legumes, green leafy vegetables), B12 (fish, pork, eggs, milk), C (raw fruits and vegetables), D (salmon, sardines, herrings, egg yolks, organ meats), Calcium (milk, almonds, green leafy vegetables, shellfish), Magnesium (seafood, whole grains, dark green vegetables, nuts), Protein (lean meat, fish, poultry, soybeans, eggs, milk, whole grains)

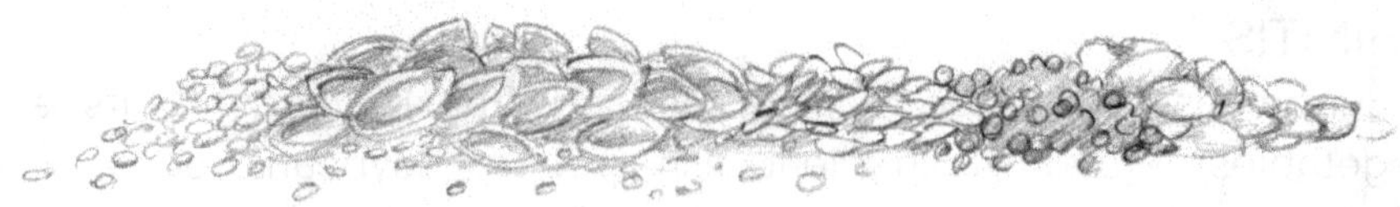

SINUSITIS

A (unprocessed orange vegetables and fruits), B group (whole grains i.e. whole or ground wheat, whole or ground brown rice), C (raw fruits and vegetables), E (cold-pressed vegetable oils, egg, wheat germ, sweet potato, leaf vegetables), Calcium (milk, almonds, green leafy vegetables, shellfish), Potassium (lean meats, whole grains, vegetables, dried fruits, legumes, sunflower seeds, avocados, cantaloupes, plantains), Zinc (pumpkin seeds, sunflower seeds, seafood, mushrooms, soybeans, oysters, herring, eggs, wheat germ, lean meats), Protein (lean meat, fish, poultry, soybeans, eggs, milk, whole grains)

SKIN PROBLEMS

BITES, STINGS, POISONS

Vitamin C (raw fruits and vegetables) See a medical physician.

BOIL OR FURUNCLE (infected nodule)

A (unprocessed orange vegetables and fruits), C (raw fruits and vegetables), E (cold-pressed vegetable oils, egg, wheat germ, sweet potato, leaf vegetables), Zinc (including pumpkin seeds, sunflower seeds, seafood, mushrooms, soybeans, oysters, herring, eggs, wheat germ, lean meats)

CANKER SORES

B group (whole grains i.e. whole or ground wheat, whole or ground brown rice), Zinc (pumpkin seeds, sunflower seeds, seafood, mushrooms, soybeans, oysters, herring, eggs, wheat germ, lean meats), Magnesium (seafood, whole grains, dark green vegetables, nuts), B1 (whole grains, molasses, brown rice, fish, lean meats, poultry, egg yolks, sunflower seeds, pistachios, quail, pork), B2 (almonds, wild rice, venison, whole grains, molasses, egg yolks, legumes, nuts), Iron (lean meats, fish, poultry, cherry juice, green leafy vegetables, dried fruits), Folic Acid (dark green leafy vegetables, root vegetables, whole grains, oysters, salmon, milk), B12 (fish, pork, eggs, milk), plain natural yogurt

MOUTH

A (unprocessed orange vegetables and fruits), D (salmon, sardines, herrings, egg yolks, organ meats), B group (whole grains i.e. whole or ground wheat, whole or ground brown rice), and water filtered, detoxified rainwater

CARBUNCLE

A (unprocessed orange vegetables and fruits), D (salmon, sardines, herrings, egg yolks, organ meats), C (raw fruits and vegetables). With fever, include E (cold-pressed vegetable oils, egg, wheat germ, sweet potato, leaf vegetables) and nutrients.

DRY SKIN

A (unprocessed orange vegetables and fruits), C (raw fruits and vegetables), B group (whole grains i.e. whole or ground wheat, whole or ground brown rice), Pantothenic Acid (egg yolks, legumes, whole grains, wheat germ, salmon), Niacin (including peanuts, fish, lean meats, poultry, milk, rice bran)

FUNGUS INFESTATIONS

(Athlete's foot, ringworm, mouth, genitals, anus, fingers, fingernails): A (unprocessed orange vegetables and fruits), B group (whole grains i.e. whole or ground wheat, whole or ground brown rice), C (raw fruits and vegetables), plain natural yogurt

ICHTHYOSIS (patches of dry skin that turn dark and scaly)

Niacin (peanuts, fish, lean meats, poultry, milk, rice bran), B group (whole grains i.e. whole or ground wheat, whole or ground brown rice), A (unprocessed orange vegetables and fruits), C (raw fruits and vegetables)

IMPETIGO

A (unprocessed orange vegetables and fruits), C (raw fruits and vegetables), D (salmon, sardines, herrings, egg yolks, organ meats), E (cold-pressed vegetable oils, egg, wheat germ, sweet potato, leaf vegetables)

ITCHING SKIN

Iron (lean meats, fish, poultry, cherry juice, green leafy vegetables, dried fruits)

LIP PROBLEMS

B2 (almonds, wild rice, venison, whole grains, molasses, egg yolks, legumes, nuts), B6 (brown rice, pinto beans, trout, sunflower seeds, whole grains, wheat germ, legumes, green leafy vegetables), B group (whole grains i.e. whole or ground wheat, whole or ground brown rice), Folic Acid (dark green leafy vegetables, root vegetables, whole grains, oysters, salmon, milk), Pantothenic Acid (egg yolks, legumes, whole grains, wheat germ, salmon), Unsaturated fatty acids (vegetable oils, sunflower seeds), and filtered, detoxified rainwater

LUPUS ERYTHEMATOSUS

B group (whole grains i.e. whole or ground wheat, whole or ground brown rice), E (cold-pressed vegetable oils, egg, wheat germ, sweet potato, leaf vegetables), Pantothenic Acid (egg yolks, legumes, whole grains, wheat germ, salmon), Manganese (whole grains, green leafy vegetables, legumes, nuts, pineapple, egg yolks, lima beans, sunflower seeds, tapioca, blackberries)

OILY SKIN

B2 (almonds, wild rice, venison, whole grains, molasses, egg yolks, legumes, nuts), B group (whole grains i.e. whole or ground wheat, whole or ground brown rice)

PIGMENTATION

A (unprocessed orange vegetables and fruits), B group (whole grains i.e. whole or ground wheat, whole or ground brown rice), C (raw fruits and vegetables), D (salmon, sardines, herrings, egg yolks, organ meats), E (cold-pressed vegetable oils, egg, wheat germ, sweet potato, leaf vegetables). Folic Acid (dark green vegetables, root vegetables, whole grains, oysters, salmon, milk), Pantothenic Acid (egg yolks, legumes, whole grains, wheat germ, salmon) and/or Niacin (peanuts, fish, lean meats, poultry, milk, rice bran)

PRICKLY HEAT

C (raw fruits and vegetables)

PURPURA

E (cold-pressed vegetable oils, egg, wheat germ, sweet potato, leaf vegetables)

SCARS

E (cold-pressed vegetable oils, egg, wheat germ, sweet potato, leaf vegetables)

DUPUYTREN'S CONTRACTURE AND PEYRONIE'S DISEASE

E (wheat germ, egg, sweet potato, leaf vegetables, cold-pressed vegetable oils)

KELOIDS

E (cold-pressed vegetable oils, egg, wheat germ, sweet potato, leaf vegetables), Zinc (pumpkin seeds, sunflower seeds, seafood, mushrooms, soybeans, oysters, herring, eggs, wheat germ, lean meats)

STRETCH MARKS

E (cold-pressed vegetable oils, egg, wheat germ, sweet potato, leaf vegetables, cucumber), B group (whole grains i.e. whole or ground wheat, whole or ground brown rice), Pantothenic Acid (egg yolks, legumes, whole grains, wheat germ, salmon), Zinc (pumpkin seeds, sunflower seeds, seafood, mushrooms, soybeans, oysters, herring, eggs, wheat germ, lean meats), C (raw fruits and vegetables)

ULCERS (Skin)

E (cold-pressed vegetable oils, egg, wheat germ, sweet potato, leaf vegetables) and topically, C (raw fruits and vegetables), Pantothenic Acid (egg yolks, legumes, whole grains, wheat germ, salmon), Folic Acid (dark green vegetables, root vegetables, whole grains, oysters, salmon, milk), Unsaturated Fatty Acids (vegetable oils, sunflower seeds)

VITILIGO

B Group (whole grains i.e. whole or ground wheat, whole or ground brown rice), Pantothenic Acid (egg yolks, legumes, whole grains, wheat germ, salmon), PABA (wheat germ, plain natural yogurt, molasses, green leafy vegetables), B6 (brown rice, pinto beans, trout, sunflower seeds, whole grains, wheat germ, legumes, green leafy vegetables, C (raw fruits and vegetables), Zinc (pumpkin seeds, sunflower seeds, seafood, mushrooms, soybeans, oysters, herring, eggs, wheat germ, lean meats), Manganese (whole grains, green leafy vegetables, legumes, nuts, pineapple, egg yolks, lima beans, sunflower seeds, tapioca, blackberries)

WARTS

E (cold-pressed vegetable oils, egg, wheat germ, sweet potato, leaf vegetables)

WRINKLES

A (unprocessed orange vegetables and fruits), B1 (whole grains, molasses, brown rice, fish, lean meats, poultry, egg yolks, sunflower seeds, pistachios, quail, pork), C (raw fruits and vegetables), E (cold-pressed vegetable oils, egg, wheat germ, sweet potato, leaf vegetables, cucumber), Zinc (pumpkin seeds, sunflower seeds, seafood, mushrooms, soybeans, oysters, herring, eggs, wheat germ, lean meats), Selenium (tuna, herring, wheat germ, wheat bran, whole grains, sesame seeds)

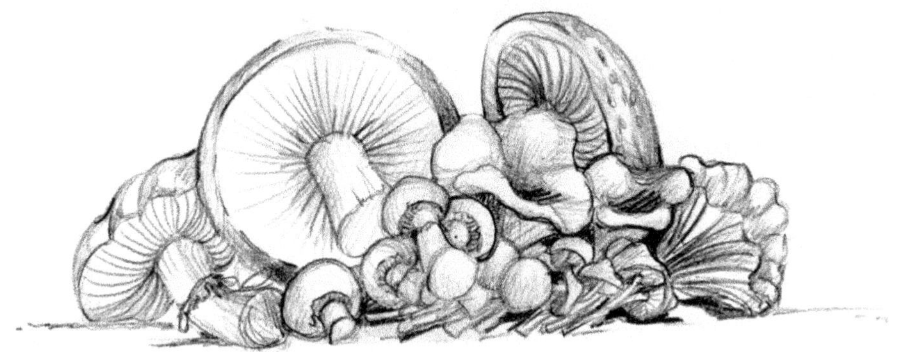

STRESS

A (unprocessed orange vegetables and fruits), B group (whole grains i.e. whole or ground wheat, whole or ground brown rice), B1 (whole grains, molasses, brown rice, fish, lean meats, poultry, egg yolks, sunflower seeds, pistachios, quail, pork), B2 (almonds, wild rice, venison, whole grains, molasses, egg yolks, legumes, nuts), B6 (brown rice, pinto beans, trout, sunflower seeds, whole grains, wheat germ, legumes, green leafy vegetables, B12 (fish, pork, eggs, milk), Biotin (egg yolks, unpolished rice, whole grains, sardines, legumes), Choline (egg yolks, wheat germ, soybeans, fish, legumes), Folic Acid (dark green leafy vegetables), root vegetables, whole grains, oysters, salmon, milk), Inositol (whole grains, citrus fruits, molasses, lean meats, milk, nuts. vegetables), Niacin (peanuts, fish, lean meats, poultry, milk, rice bran), PABA (wheat germ, plain natural yogurt, molasses, green leafy vegetables), C (raw fruits and vegetables), D (salmon, sardines, herrings, egg yolks, organ meats), E (cold-pressed vegetable oils, egg, wheat germ, sweet potato, leaf vegetables), Calcium (milk, almonds, green leafy vegetables, shellfish), Chromium (grapes, raisins, corn oil, clams, whole grains), Copper (seafood, nuts, legumes, molasses, raisins), Iodine (seafood, kelp), Iron (lean meats, fish, poultry, cherry juice, green leafy vegetables, dried fruits), Magnesium (seafood, whole grains, dark green vegetables, nuts), Manganese (whole grains, green leafy vegetables, legumes, nuts, pineapple, egg yolks, lima beans, sunflower seeds, tapioca, blackberries), Phosphorus (fish, lean meats, poultry, eggs, milk, nuts, whole grains), Potassium (lean meats, whole grains, vegetables, dried fruits, legumes, sunflower seeds, avocados, cantaloupes, plantains), Selenium (tuna, herring, wheat germ, wheat bran, whole grains, sesame seeds), Zinc (pumpkin seeds, sunflower seeds, seafood, mushrooms, soybeans, oysters, herring, eggs, wheat germ, lean meats), Carbohydrate (whole grains, fruits, vegetables), Fat (vegetable oils, butter, whole milk, nuts, seeds), Protein (lean meat, fish, poultry, soybeans, eggs, milk, whole grains)

STROKE

B group (including whole grains i.e. whole or ground wheat, whole or ground brown rice), Choline (egg yolks, wheat germ, soybeans, fish, legumes), Inositol (whole grains, citrus fruits, molasses, lean meats, milk, nuts, vegetables), C (raw fruits and vegetables), E (cold-pressed vegetable oils, egg, wheat germ, sweet potato, leaf vegetables), Bioflavonoids (citrus fruits, fruits, blackcurrants, buckwheat), Potassium (lean meats, whole grains, vegetables, dried fruits, legumes, sunflower seeds, avocados, cantaloupes, plantains), Selenium (tuna, herring, wheat germ, vegetables, dried fruits, legumes, sunflower seeds), Zinc (pumpkin seeds, sunflower seeds, seafood, mushrooms, soybeans, oysters, herring, eggs, wheat germ, lean meats), Protein (lean meat, fish, poultry, soybeans, eggs, milk, whole grains)

SUNBURN

A (unprocessed orange vegetables and fruits), B group (whole grains i.e. whole or ground wheat, whole or ground brown rice), B6 (brown rice, pinto beans, trout, sunflower seeds, whole grains, wheat germ, legumes, green leafy vegetables), PABA (wheat germ, plain natural yogurt, molasses, green leafy vegetables), C (raw fruits and vegetables), E (cold-pressed vegetable oils, egg, wheat germ, sweet potato, leaf vegetables, cucumber), Calcium (milk, almonds, green leafy vegetables, shellfish), Zinc (pumpkin seeds, sunflower seeds, seafood, mushrooms, soybeans, oysters, herring, eggs, wheat germ, lean meats)

SWOLLEN GLANDS

A (unprocessed orange vegetables and fruits), B group (whole grains i.e. whole or ground wheat, whole or ground brown rice), B6 (brown rice, pinto beans, trout, sunflower seeds, whole grains, wheat germ, legumes, green leafy vegetables), Pantothenic Acid (egg yolks, legumes, whole grains, wheat germ, salmon), C (raw fruits and vegetables), Protein (lean meat, fish, poultry, soybeans, eggs, milk, whole grains), and filtered, detoxified rainwater

TETANY

Magnesium (crustaceans, nuts, whole grains, dark green vegetables)

TICS, TREMORS, AND TWITCHES

Magnesium (seafood, whole grains, dark-green vegetables, nuts), Potassium (lean meats, whole grains, vegetables, dried fruits, legumes, sunflower seeds, avocados, cantaloupes, plantains), B group (whole grains i.e. whole or ground wheat, whole or ground brown rice), B6 (brown rice, pinto beans, trout, sunflower seeds, whole grains, wheat germ, legumes, green leafy vegetables), B12 (fish, pork, eggs, milk), Niacin (peanuts, fish, lean meats, poultry, milk, rice bran)

TONSILLITIS

A (unprocessed orange vegetables and fruits), B group (whole grains i.e. whole or ground wheat, whole or ground brown rice), B2 (almonds, wild rice, venison, whole grains, molasses, egg yolks, legumes, nuts), B6 (brown rice, pinto beans, trout, sunflower seeds, whole grains, wheat germ, legumes, green leafy vegetables), Folic Acid (dark green leafy vegetables, root vegetables, whole grains, oysters, salmon, milk), Pantothenic Acid (egg yolks, legumes, whole grains, wheat germ, salmon), C (raw fruits and vegetables), D (salmon, sardines, herrings, egg yolks, organ meats), E (cold-pressed vegetable oils, egg, wheat germ, sweet potato, leaf vegetables), Protein (lean meat, fish, poultry, soybeans, eggs, milk, whole grains)

TOOTH AND GUM DISORDERS

A (unprocessed orange vegetables and fruits), B6 (brown rice, pinto beans, trout, sunflower seeds, whole grains, wheat germ, legumes, green leafy vegetables), Niacin (peanuts, fish, lean meats, poultry, milk, rice bran), C (raw fruits and vegetables), D (salmon, sardines, herrings, egg yolks, organ meats), Bioflavonoids (citrus fruits, fruits, blackcurrants, buckwheat), Calcium (milk, almonds, green leafy vegetables, shellfish), Copper (seafood, nuts, legumes, molasses, raisins), Fluorine (sea foods, cheese, lean meat, tea), Iron (lean meats, eggs, fish, poultry, molasses, cherry juice, green leafy vegetables, dried fruits), Magnesium (seafood, whole grains, dark green vegetables, nuts), Manganese (whole grains, green leafy vegetables, legumes, nuts, pineapple, egg yolks, lima beans, sunflower seeds, tapioca, blackberries), Phosphorus (fish, lean meats, poultry, eggs, milk, nuts, whole grains), Potassium (lean meats, whole grains, vegetables, dried fruits, legumes, sunflower seeds, avocados, cantaloupes, plantains), Sodium (seafood, kelp), Zinc (pumpkin seeds, sunflower seeds, seafood, mushrooms, soybeans, oysters, herring, eggs, wheat germ, lean meats), Protein (lean meat, fish, poultry, soybeans, eggs, milk, whole grains), Unsaturated Fatty Acids 1 - 2tbsp (vegetable oils, sunflower seeds)

TUBERCULOSIS

A (unprocessed orange vegetables and fruits), B group (whole grains i.e. whole or ground wheat, whole or ground brown rice), B6 (brown rice, pinto beans, trout, sunflower seeds, whole grains, wheat germ, legumes, green leafy vegetables), D (salmon, sardines, herrings, egg yolks, organ meats), Calcium (milk, almonds, green leafy vegetables, shellfish), Iron (lean meats, fish, poultry, cherry juice, green leafy vegetables, dried fruits), Phosphorus (fish, lean meats, poultry, eggs, milk, nuts, whole grains), Zinc (pumpkin seeds, sunflower seeds, seafood, mushrooms, soybeans, oysters, herring, eggs, wheat germ, lean meats), Manganese (whole grains, green leafy vegetables, legumes, nuts, pineapple, egg yolks, lima beans, sunflower seeds, tapioca, blackberries), Protein (lean meat, fish, poultry, soybeans, eggs, milk, whole grains)

ULCER

A (unprocessed orange vegetables and fruits), B group (whole grains i.e. whole or ground wheat, whole or ground brown rice), B2 (almonds, wild rice, venison, whole grains, molasses, egg yolks, legumes, nuts), B6 (brown rice, pinto beans, trout, sunflower seeds, whole grains, wheat germ, legumes, green leafy vegetables), B12 (fish, pork, eggs, milk), Choline (egg yolks, wheat germ, soybeans, fish, legumes), Folic Acid (dark-green leafy vegetables, root vegetables, whole grains, oysters, salmon, milk), Pantothenic Acid (egg yolks, legumes, whole grains, wheat germ, salmon), C (raw fruits and vegetables), D (salmon, sardines, herrings, egg yolks, organ meats), E (cold-pressed vegetable oils, egg, wheat germ, sweet potato, leaf vegetables), K (green leafy vegetables, egg yolks, safflower oil, molasses, cauliflower, soybeans), Bioflavonoids (citrus fruits, fruits, blackcurrants, buckwheat), Calcium (milk, almonds, green leafy vegetables, shellfish), Iron (lean meats, fish, poultry, cherry juice, green leafy vegetables, dried fruits), Manganese (whole grains, green leafy vegetables, legumes, nuts, pineapple, egg yolks, lima beans, sunflower seeds, tapioca, blackberries), Zinc (pumpkin seeds, sunflower seeds, seafood, mushrooms, soybeans, oysters, herring, eggs, wheat germ, lean meats), Protein (lean meat, fish, poultry, soybeans, eggs, milk, whole grains), plain natural yogurt, Unsaturated fatty acids (vegetable oils, sunflower seeds)

UNDERWEIGHT

B group (whole grains i.e. whole or ground wheat, whole or ground brown rice), Protein (lean meat, fish, poultry, soybean, eggs, milk, whole grains), Unsaturated fatty acids (vegetable oils, sunflower seeds)

VAGINITIS

A (unprocessed orange vegetables and fruits), B group (whole grains i.e. whole or ground wheat, whole or ground brown rice), B2 (almonds, wild rice, venison, whole grains, molasses, egg yolks, legumes, nuts), B6 (brown rice, pinto beans, trout, sunflower seeds, whole grains, wheat germ, legumes, green leafy vegetables), D (salmon, sardines, herrings, egg yolks, organ meats), E (cold-pressed vegetable oils, egg, wheat germ, sweet potato, leaf vegetables, cucumber), Protein (lean meat, fish, poultry, soybean, eggs, milk, whole grains), plain natural yogurt

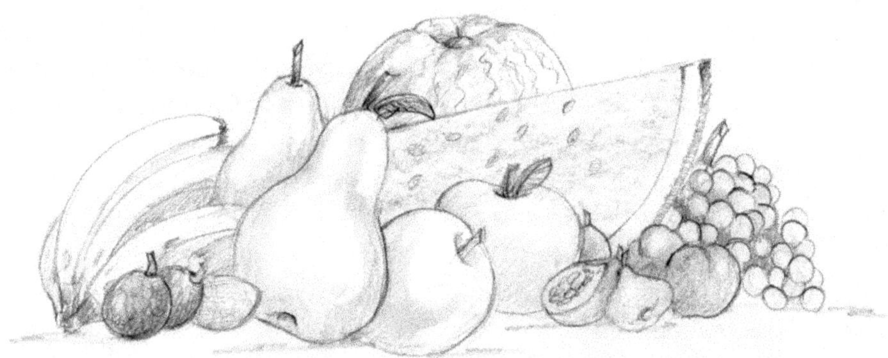

VARICOSE VEINS

B group (whole grains i.e. whole or ground wheat, whole or ground brown rice), C (raw fruits and vegetables), E (cold-pressed vegetable oils, egg, wheat germ, sweet potato, leaf vegetables), Bioflavonoids (citrus fruits, fruits, blackcurrants, buckwheat), Protein (lean meat, fish, poultry, soybeans, eggs, milk, whole grains), Unsaturated fatty acids (vegetable oils, sunflower seeds)

VENEREAL DISEASE

B group (whole grains i.e. whole or ground wheat, whole or ground brown rice), Protein (lean meat, fish, poultry, soybeans, eggs, milk, whole grains), plain natural yogurt

WERNICKE'S ENCEPHALOPATHY

B1 (whole grains, molasses, brown rice, fish, lean meats, poultry, egg yolks, sunflower seeds, pistachios, quail, pork), Magnesium (seafood, whole grains, dark green vegetables, nuts), Phosphorus (fish, lean meat, poultry, eggs, milk, nuts, whole grains)

WILSON'S DISEASE

Zinc (pumpkin seeds, sunflower seeds, seafood, mushrooms, soybeans, oysters, herring, eggs, wheat germ, lean meats), Calcium (milk, almonds, green leafy vegetables, shellfish), Magnesium (seafood, whole grains, dark green vegetables, nuts)

XEROPHTHALMIA

A (unprocessed orange vegetables and fruits), B group (whole grains i.e. whole or ground wheat, whole or ground brown rice), B1 (whole grains, molasses, brown rice, lean meats, fish, poultry, egg yolks, sunflower seeds, pistachios, quail, pork), B2 (almonds, wild rice, venison, whole grains, molasses, egg yolks, legumes, nuts), B6 (brown rice, pinto beans, trout, sunflower seeds, whole grains, wheat germ, legumes, green leafy vegetables), Niacin (peanuts, fish, lean meats, poultry, milk, rice bran), Pantothenic Acid (egg yolks, legumes, whole grains, wheat germ, salmon), C (raw fruits and vegetables), Bioflavonoids (citrus fruits, fruits, blackcurrants, buckwheat), D (salmon, sardines, herrings, egg yolks, organ meats), E (cold-pressed vegetable oils, egg, wheat germ, sweet potato, leaf vegetables), Calcium (milk, almonds, green leafy vegetables, shellfish), Magnesium (seafood, whole grains, dark green vegetables, nuts), Zinc (pumpkin seeds, sunflower seeds, seafood, mushrooms, soybeans, oysters, herring, eggs, wheat germ, lean meats), Protein (lean meat, fish, poultry, soybeans, eggs, milk, whole grains), Unsaturated fatty acids (vegetable oils, sunflower seeds), and filtered, detoxified rainwater
Symptoms: Dry sandy eyes with thick white mucosa

XEROSTOMIA

A (unprocessed orange vegetables and fruits), B group (whole grains i.e. whole or ground wheat, whole or ground brown rice), B2 (whole grains, egg yolks, legumes, nuts), B6 (lean meats, whole grains, wheat germ, legumes, green leafy vegetables), B12 (fish, pork, eggs, low salt cheese, milk), Folic Acid (dark-green vegetables, root vegetables, whole grains, oysters, salmon, milk), Inositol (whole grains, citrus fruits, meat, milk, nuts, vegetables), Niacin (peanuts, rice bran, trout, salmon, rabbit, pheasant, quail), PABA (wheat germ, yogurt, green leafy vegetables. molasses), Pantothenic Acid (egg yolks, legumes, whole grains, wheat germ, salmon), C (raw fruits and vegetables), D (salmon, sardines, herrings, egg yolks, organ meats), E (cold-pressed vegetable oils, eggs, wheat germ), Unsaturated Fatty Acids (vegetable oils, sunflower seeds), Bioflavonoids (unprocessed citrus fruits, fruits, blackcurrants, buckwheat), Calcium (skim milk, green leafy vegetables, shellfish), Copper (seafood, nuts, legumes, raisins), Iodine (seafood, kelp), Magnesium (seafood, whole grains, dark green vegetables, nuts), Manganese (whole grains, green leafy vegetables, legumes, nuts, pineapple, egg yolk), Phosphorus (fish, lean meat, poultry, eggs, milk, nuts, whole grains), Potassium (lean meats, whole grains, vegetables, dried fruits, legumes, sunflower seeds), Selenium (tuna, herring, wheat germ, wheat bran, whole grains, sesame seeds), Sulphur (fish, red peppers, garlic, onions, eggs, lean meats, cabbage, brussel sprouts, horseradish), Protein (meat, fish, poultry, soybeans, eggs, milk, whole grains), Zinc (pumpkin seeds, sunflower seeds, seafood, mushrooms, soybeans, oysters, herring, eggs, wheat germ, lean meat), E (cold-pressed oils, eggs, wheat germ, sweet potato, leafy vegetables) Symptoms: Dryness of mouth that can lead to dental decay, gingivitis and difficulty chewing and swallowing. Most Probable Cause: Accumulation of fluid in the membrane lining the joints, and inflammation of surrounding tissues

YAWNING

Fresh air, deep breathing

ZINC DEFICIENCY

Zinc (pumpkin seeds, sunflower seeds, seafood, mushrooms, soybeans, oysters, herring, eggs, wheat germ, lean meats); Deficiency can be caused by a diet high in unrefined cereal and unleavened bread (Ref: Mahan & Escott-Stump, 1996, Book, *Krause's Food, Nutrition & Diet*, (Online), Available: www.amazon.com/)

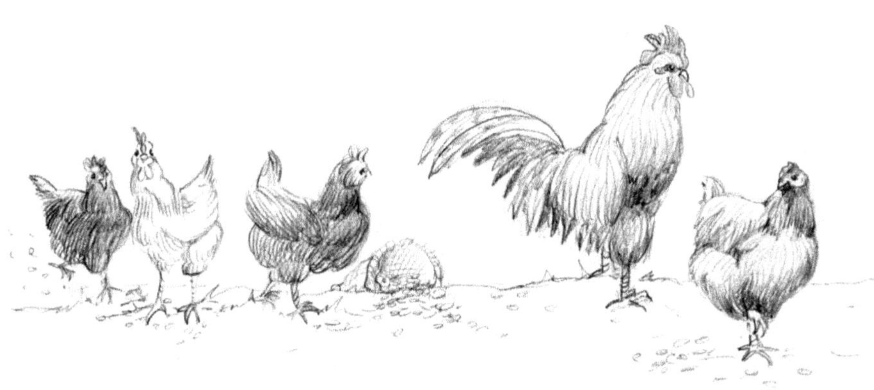

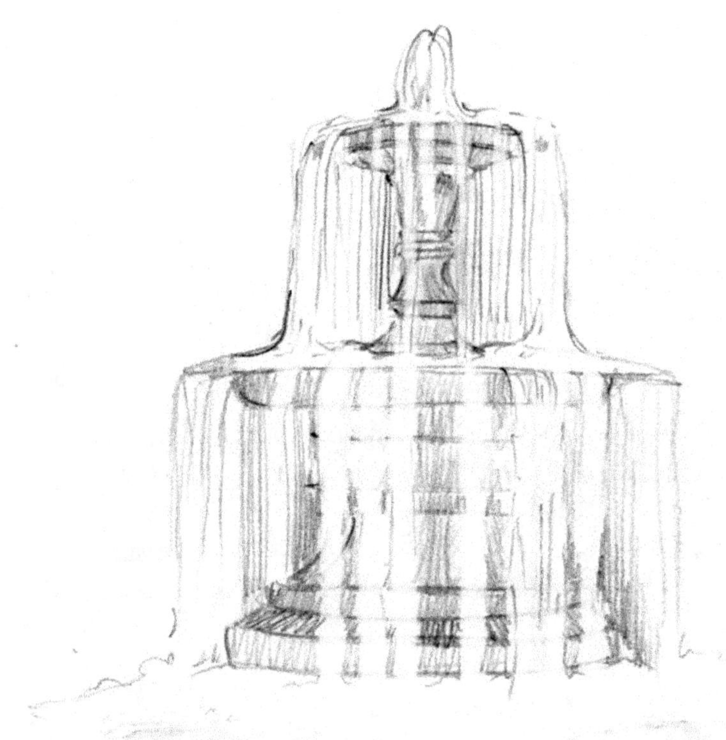

PART 3

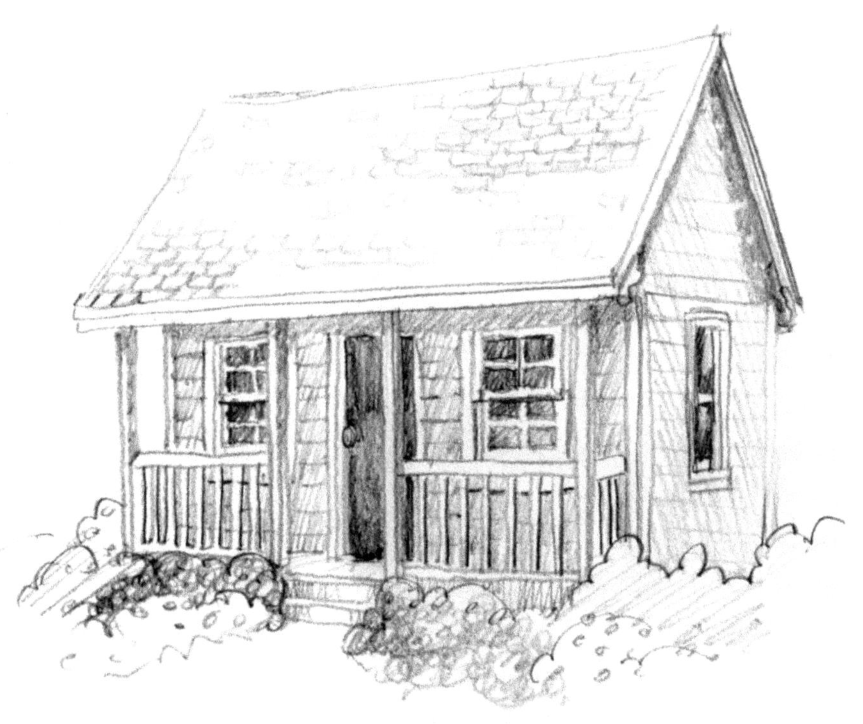

The Author

Born 16-10-1954, I grew up on a farm near Monduran, Yandaran, about one hour's drive north of Bundaberg. The air and was ever so clean and rainwater was such a Divine substance that every drop was precious and treated accordingly. Life there as settlers was tough and very hard, laborious work. I helped my parents in clearing land for fodder crops to feed dairy and beef cattle, planting, fertilizing with nutrients to produce luscious growth, along with planting corn to feed pigs and poultry, placing rows of irrigation pipes for daily watering from dams until plants matured, then setting up portable fences to slow the cattle's over-indulgence amidst their ecstasy in green. Cattle's eating habits can be similar to dogs. They keep eating until it is too late to feel comfortable then suffer with stomach and abdominal discomfort for a day or more.

Timber was cut from and sawn on the property in 1960 that built the new family homestead, sheds, pigs' pens, breeding and poultry houses, holding yards, cattle crush and ramps. Milk from the dairy cows was separated on the farm and the cream was railed to Bundaberg for the manufacture of naturally golden-coloured butter. Beef cattle and white pigs were bred for market. Also on this farm were about twenty hens, lots of chickens (reared by the few bantam hens - a small breed of domestic fowl that hid their eggs away from the nesting boxes and returned with about a dozen chickens following), roosters (one ended up in the pot on most Sundays for lunch that my mother turned into a delicious soup), a few turkeys, three dogs, large tabby farm cat, horses for mustering purposes as the dairy and beef cattle needed (at the time) to be dipped in an arsenic and water mixture to kill ticks and to help them be freed of the blood-sucking vermin approximately every three weeks, and a large cage of melodious king parrots, galahs and cockatoos which my step-brother caught to stop them from ruining freshly planted crops. Friends would visit and were often given a bird to take home as a pet.

If an animal fell ill it was given the very best of care because this was our family's livelihood. We needed to see an animal well again due to the immense workload in feeding each creature. The major reason why an animal became dis-eased was because of a nutritional deficiency. This too is what mainly happens in the human race.

Following many years of various ailments, which were always treated through the normal medical system, it appeared that there was a better and more long-term cure for these.

A long trail of unnecessary excruciating operations, addictive prescribed narcotics, x-rays and tests is forever in the past, never to be repeated, having learned better ways to live.

With my father going to the 'other side' after his human existence and the concerns of losing family members before their average three score and ten years, this driving force inside wanted to know why. After being divinely guided to study massage therapy, I left my job as tour desk operator at a beautiful beach resort and the rest is history in *The Australian Massage*, *The Australian Advanced and Metaphysical Massage* and *Simple Foods to Heal Your Body*.

With seventeen years of suffering from skin ailments behind me, reality came when I was refused skin analysis and yet laboratories were happy to perform other tests looking for certain types of fungi. I was told that the only way the Australian medical system allowed for the continuous thick layers of peeling skin to be analysed was during an autopsy. No one had advised them that I wasn't planning on leaving this body yet! This was not acceptable so I called forensic. Being informed by a member of the forensic department that these tests would cost many thousands of dollars and myself not having the thousands of dollars required to have tests that I asked for to be carried out, I prayed for help.

Every afternoon I applied guided meditation for healing and on this particular day I asked for help to escape from the daily pain and bring forth the answers necessary to heal permanently. A thick, crusted coating used to peel from my hands daily and at times with metal flecks of silver, copper, black and gold colours attached which were, I believe, fragments of metal that fell into cans upon opening and were swallowed along with other foreign material from some pre-packaged food items. Cracks became so deep on my hands that two metacarpal bones were exposed due to the physically demanding work I was performing hence the wearing of surgical gloves became a necessity. I also believe that sharp, embedded, foreign objects can be the growing point for a cyst.

An arsenic mixture I used to blend and stir into the cattle dip that splashed only slightly but enough to be absorbed into my skin may have contributed. A lethal mixture that was injected into wattle tree suckers to stop their continual taking over of cleared ground with the occasional drop landing onto my skin and being absorbed may have contributed.

Sucking in toxic smoke from lit cigarettes contributed until 1993 after a meditation 'told' me that I only sucked on cigarettes because I was still following the leader - my father who was role model and had spiritually left this planet in 1984!

Excess sugar intake contributed due to very high internal acid levels. The fear of failure was intense so this too contributed to being 'thin skinned.' I can go on and on (however I have already written about many reasons for specific ailments) yet most of these problems came about due to an extremely low self-esteem and poor eating habits.

I was born extremely confident however somewhere during my childhood, my well-meaning parents passed on their insecure feelings and taught me feelings of inadequacy and fear.

Self-love is the healing process that assists on our pathway to a more healthy life. Access to health is readily available because we desire more time and energy for our life's purpose while enjoying living on this planet.

After opening my heart freely during that meditation in 1993 the answers flowed in. Photographs of serious skin problems serve as a reminder of what poor nutrition, poisons and specific chemicals touching the skin and lungs, poor indoor air quality and electromagnetic fields radiating from electrical appliances (and especially from old computer systems and phones emitting high electromagnetic fields - discovered when learning Modern Feng Shui at an Australian Government recognised college) can do.

Nutritious food, finely filtered rain water and positive re-enforcements all make way for our future generations' prosperity. There are a lot of people who would benefit more in their lives by learning communication skills as these were certainly lacking in the household where I grew up. Louise Hay's book, *You Can Heal Your Life* is one of the best I know of to begin with for clearing up past negative experiences and is listed under *References*.

To play with our earth, sea, sun and air are the greatest gifts from above. We are given these presents to create our lives any way we choose. We are blessed with all required for our survival. Each of us can make a living from that which a country gives to us - when we nurture these gifts for the betterment of human beings on this planet. Success doesn't come overnight but the power to be successful can. With a strong belief in oneself, setting out a nine year growth plan and getting started on it calls for many a celebration along the way.

After many years of studies and practice, the passing of my sister in 1998 gave the final motivation to apply for registration of my course which I knew worked for so many people: myself, patients, students and practitioners for over ten years. On the 8th of February 1999 I was awarded a Certificate of Accreditation for my *Course in Natural Health*, a nationally recognised training product which I believed would assist in the spreading of the knowledge on how to become healthy so we could all live healthier ever after. This I ceased in 2004 to concentrate more on marketing my favourite commodity - rainwater, knowing it has the superior ability to move through the cells which continually need cleansing, moving nutrients in and wastes out, returning the body to its natural vital state.

I am hopeful that the sharing of *Simple Foods to Heal Your* Body can help people be saved from physical pain, even in a small way. There are many good books written on nutrition. Each one can give an enlightening broader picture for even more understanding.

I have been singing the joys of *RAINFOREST DEW™*, Australia's premium bottled rainwater from the pristine rainforest regions of Far North Queensland since 1995 because it is packed with energising oxygen and tastes so pure with no added chlorine or metals. Through all of my nutrition studies I discovered that chlorine in drinking water destroys vitamin E and can damage capillaries. Vitamin E has a positive effect on the reproductive organs. Vitamin E also assists in eliminating body odour, headaches and certain menstrual problems to name a few. Drinking unfiltered, chlorinated water calls for the addition of foods that contain vitamin E.

RAINFOREST DEW™ rainwater is also low in bicarbonate and is welcomed in the blood stream. What has this got to do with water which the average human body is 70% of? During twenty-five years in Practice many of the people I treated suffered with back and ligaments problems. During my years of studying nutrition I discovered that excessive bicarbonate in the system seriously depletes the body of vitamin C. Vitamin C helps give the much-needed elasticity to the spinal discs and ligaments. Bicarbonate opposes vitamin C therefore destroying it. Calcium and magnesium together also play a large role and so too do many other nutrients as you now know.

Learning more about each nutrient's special place in the human body and what one and all can do is a good investment for our future. Maintaining a regular nutritional update is wise when healing a serious ailment.

Raw sprouts, raw salads and raw fruits increase the spirit of liveliness in the body. Fish, poultry, lean meats, dairy, eggs, nuts, and whole grains can supply extra energy for daily bodily activities that incorporate moderate to heavy exercise and less of these for activities that are light and leisurely. Known food allergies are always deleted from any daily intake.

Where I am at today is working on what I love, helping people to be pain free naturally, happily promoting Mother Nature's rainwater, whilst placing more emphasis on my left side and will be for the remainder of this life, knowing it took over fifty years before this body said, "Enough is enough!" Had I have followed direction from a karate master many years ago with regards to bodily balance my hip joint would have more supporting cartilage and the left side would also be as strong and balanced. By putting my 'best' foot forward the body's right side, from excessive weight-bearing use increased the size of the right foot, leg and arm to name the most predominant. It's no wonder there are so many joint replacements being performed these days.

I also encouraged my body to come to terms more quickly with this greater plan of well-being by regularly listening to guided, positive, body affirmations in meditation and in song. My body cells responded joyously and loved this journey as they continually changed for the better. Positive, guided meditation has worked miracles in my life since 1989 so I decided to create a few CDs with my own guided meditations and an easy listening CD with the most loving life affirmations (the gift to creating miracles) for continual wellbeing.

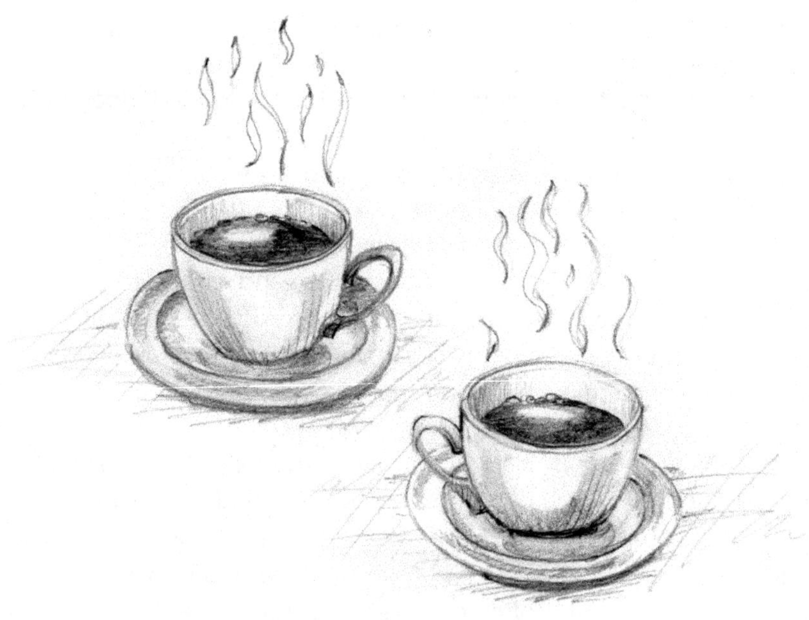

Conclusion

This book will, when used, assist the reader to improve long-term health, and will help in avoiding the excessive use of the current health industry, both in services and drugs.

It is unfortunate that the bulk of the health industry is primarily focused on treating symptoms and not the cause origins. There are many examples of individuals needlessly suffering when most ailments are controllable by a nutritious diet, exercise, meditation and a more safely built environment. According to Dr. Campbell, 1972 even crippling arthritis can be reversed if the diet is changed before pain becomes constant, and this is with a raw food diet.

Surgery is excellent for accident repairs and for conditions that have exceeded the abilities of a novice to dissolve. There are more doctors today interested in natural healing treatments, those printing their beliefs on paper and spreading good healing news as discoveries continue being proven.

The biology of and in a building where a person spends most time may also be contributing to a serious dis-ease in the body. Please see Appendix, *Modern Feng Shui Tips*. A professional consultation can determine if this is so, that also provides recommendations and remedies as are necessary.

We live in one of the best primary producing countries in the world. Farming has been flourishing for centuries. With much more effort and less 'must have now', there are golden opportunities to open more gates of plentiful produce to market for the benefit of all.

Feel the richness of your glorious country. It is abound with wealth. All it needs is your energy. By eating simple foods that heal our bodies and by being grateful every day for these, we can thrive for our country's prosperity. Life is very simple. What we give out we get back. When we feed our bodies with nourishing foods and beverages our bodies respond with vibrant energy. Whatever we love grows so by thinking happy, loving thoughts and nutritionally taking care of our bodies, these are the best ways to create a loving world and prosperity. So let's breathe in deeply, fully taking in the fresh breath of life and be nourished.

Now that you've decided to be healthy, the only reason for delay is that there is a part of you that doesn't believe that you deserve it. Are your beliefs so strong that they overpower your new positive goal, "I am healthy"? Many of us were such obedient children that we willingly accepted our parents' beliefs about life. Many people continue to operate under them for the rest of their lives. My parents knew very little about health however they knew plenty about basic survival and how to achieve growth on the land with lots of toil of which I am grateful. If my parents did know a lot about health I wouldn't have discovered the answers I have just written about.

Learning a new process has many setbacks and it is okay to make mistakes during this new learning phase. It will become easier with persistence. Every time you become aware of a setback, you can thank your intelligent brain for acknowledging, and then let it go out of your life. If the setback returns, thank your brain again and politely escort the setback out of your life again. Continue to do so until it is gone forever. The Universal laws of attraction are waiting for you to be healed. You may like to begin with this easy positive affirmation, "I lovingly take care of my body now so I can look forward to a healthy old age."

Once again, if you are suffering with any ailment and are serious about being healthier see a practitioner such as natural nutritionist, naturopath, and/or kinesiologist and commence or accelerate your journey to a healthier way in life.

Simply by enjoying a healthy way of living you will also be serving your country and saving it from the escalating expenditure for impoverished health. By lovingly working towards healing with a more permanent and positive outcome for everyone's future your body will enjoy this change immensely and so too will your country fellow beings who are all working towards your better health. It is never too late to have a happy life. Smile more and share the joy of living.

APPENDIX

Brief Introduction to Feng Shui

Contemporary and Traditional Feng Shui is all about your space and what is within that space influences every aspect of your life. Because ancient Chinese scholars observed nature thoroughly, they noticed that everything happens in cycles. There are seasons, weather patterns, moon phases, day, night and human life. The five elements of fire, earth, metal, water, and wood represent a model of our Universe, cyclical and forever changing.

If you observe the Sheng Cycle you will see how each element in the circle represents the growth cycle. Each element receives energy from the one prior and gives energy to the next, in a clockwise direction. At closer observation, by following the inner arrows you will notice how each element controls another. These are the ways of Mother Nature and we use her for our growth and understanding of life.

In Traditional Chinese Medicine fire represents summer which is heat. The colour is red and relates to the heart and circulatory system. Cool water is recommended to reduce the heat because water can control fire. A reduction in red meats and chilli may be recommended to reduce heart problems. Excessive heat (fire) may attack the air (metal). Metal represents autumn, dryness in the air and also relates to the lungs. Another example you may like to consider: Wood represents spring and winds. The colour is green and relates to the liver and gallbladder. Excess of the wood element may attack the earth element. Earth represents late summer or tropical monsoon summer, dampness and humidity and relates to the digestive organs. When we are angry or frustrated we may lose our appetite and this may lead to digestive problems, including nausea. Do you see a pattern beginning to form here? If you wish to learn more about how all this comes together then please visit The Australian College of Environmental Studies website and learn from one of the best teachers in this field.

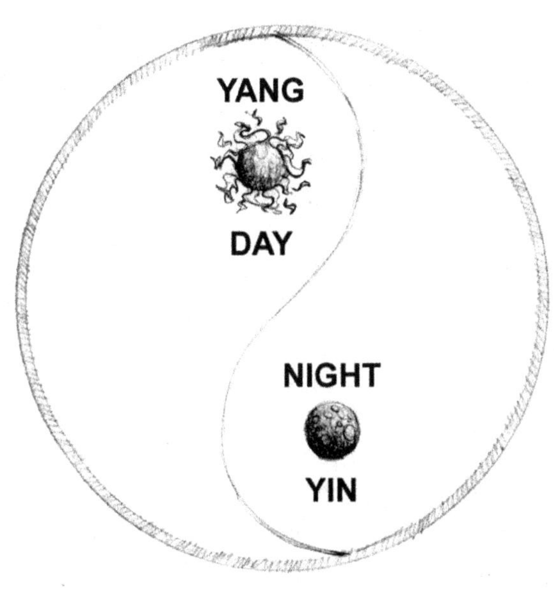

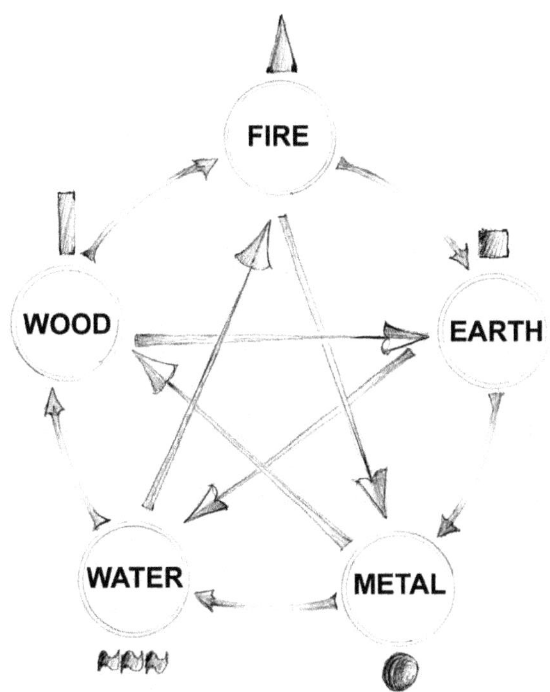

Sheng Cycle

Modern Feng Shui Tips

Remember when you last inhaled deep breaths of fresh morning garden air? Do you remember how the joyfulness spreading within your body felt? How uplifted you felt? Now imagine standing outside inhaling the fresh morning air, standing with your arms wide apart saying, "I am open and receptive to all the good and abundance in our Universe." This is similar to what it feels like when every piece of clutter leaves your home.

Everything is made up of energy and any kind of clutter within your space creates an obstacle to the smooth flow of energy. It can create stagnancy and confusion in not only your life, but other occupants' lives in the room/s too. Clutter makes one feel tired and lethargic, and can suppress emotions, depress, or keep you in the past, maybe congest your body, dull the enjoyment of life, or may make you feel ashamed and embarrassed.

Every aspect of your life is anchored energetically in your living space. Clearing clutter can completely transform your entire existence. Although your house may be very clean, neat and tidy, there are always some drawers and cupboards with things that you may feel you just cannot part with. If there are things that haven't been used during the past year or two it is now time to either use or sell these, give them away or throw out into the rubbish bin. If there are any items or gifts that were given to you by people you do not approve of today, remove those objects from your home. Clearing clutter has the effect of clearing and freeing you internally. You always feel freer and lighter, ready to take on the world.

The following information is provided to bring awareness of what else may be causing health problems that have not been able to be stopped or healed by any other means. It may be your living space that needs correcting for your body to be well. Here are a few starters to consider.

The Modern Feng Shui of the bedroom is most important as the average person sleeps around twenty two years of their life here, or you may have a favourite chair that you spend many hours sitting in each day.

It is important to be sleeping/sitting away from high electromagnetic fields (EMFs) and not sleeping/sitting over any geopathic stress (for example; underground water course, geological fault, near meter boxes) as these may lead to any of the following: loss of self-confidence and thinking faculty, ill-defined disease, sufferance with long treatment and unclear recovery, increasing heartbeat, morning fatigue (even after a good night's sleep), cold sweat, nervousness, disturbed sleep with dreams and nightmares, poor sleep, some insomnia and decline in appetite, visionary and auditory hallucinations, any illness which does not clear up despite good treatment, become ill shortly after moving into the house; wake up feeling unrefreshed or feel worse in the mornings because people are often affected by geopathic stress in bed as the body's resistance to it drops to 1/3 of normal during sleep (Jacobs, 2001).

Many behavioural and learning problems can be the result of exposure to geopathic stress. (Institute of Geopathology SA, 1993).

On average, materials such as synthetic bench tops, paints, adhesives and particleboards containing formaldehyde continually emit toxic volatile organic compounds that can contribute to air pollution in the home and workplace. Reduce these significantly with good ventilation such as open windows and plants known to absorb the toxicity.

A report by the Australian Government's National Industrial Chemicals Notification and Assessment Scheme published in 2006 states, "Breathing formaldehyde vapour can irritate the eyes and nose, which may cause burning, stinging or itching sensations, a sore throat, watery eyes, blocked sinuses, runny nose, and sneezing." Other health effects, "Formaldehyde has been shown to cause nasal cancer in animals."

After your home has been closed for a number of hours, what does it smell of when first entering? Is it appealing? What about the garage, if there is one? Are there any exhaust fumes entering the home? What does the bedroom smell of? What about the kitchen or laundry, do these need more airing? What about artificial fragrance, are there any that may cause respiratory concerns?

Reduce cleaning products and store them where they are able to off gass to the outside air. Choose cleaning products such as Abode and Biometics (www.cleanabode.com.au and www.ekobuildingbiology.com.au/biometics-safe-and-clean) that are biodegradable.

Always store food away from cleaning products or odorous materials.

Drinking finely filtered rain-water eliminates heavy metals such as lead, copper, aluminium and cadmium, chemicals such as chlorine, fluoride, pesticides, lime and UV stabilisers, also various forms of bacteria and other micro-organisms.

Light, ventilation, temperature and low noise are all-important in the study or office.

Open windows and doors when possible to maximize air flow as good ventilation is necessary for increased vitality.

I hope you enjoyed this book and may you have fun discovering new ways your home can help you to live better.

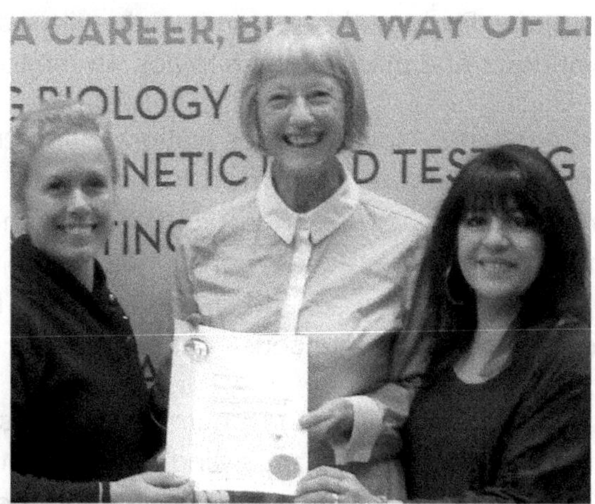

Receiving Certificate IV in Feng Shui (2014) at Australian College of Environmental Studies

Presented by Principal/Teacher Nicole Bijlsma (left) and Teacher Katina Benis (right)

REFERENCES

Australian Government's National Industrial Chemicals Notification and Assessment Scheme 2006, "Formaldehyde safety for workers Factsheet," (Online), Available: www.nicnas.gov.au/communication.publiscations/information-sheets/existing-chemical-info-sheets/formaldehyde-in-pressed-wood-products-safety-factsheet

Bachler, Kathe 1989, *Earth Radiation - The Startling Discoveries of a Dowser*, "Geopathic Stress and Children," (Online), Available: http://www.megadisc.com.au/index_files/geopathic2.htm

Bijlsma, Nicole 2010, "Certificate IV in Building Biology," Australian College of Environmental Studies, Suite 2 / 25-29 Prospect St, Box Hill, VIC, 3128, (Online), Available: www.buildingbiology.com or www.aces.edu.au

Hay, Louise L. 1987, Book, *You Can Heal Your Life*, (Online), Available: Specialist Publications, P.O. 143, Concord, NSW, 2137, Australia

Institute of Geopathology SA 1993, (Online), Available: http://geopathology-za.wikidot.com/kaethe-bachler

Jacobs, Dr Robert MRCS, LRCP 2001, "Geopathic Stress," *"If geopathic stress is natural why is it dangerous and why have we not become immune to it?" "How do you treat geopathic stress?"* (pg 3-4), (Online), Available: http://www.wholisticresearch.com.info/artshow.php3?artid=211

Minnesota Dept. of Health, 2011 Formaldehyde in Your Home, "What is Formaldehyde," Where is it found?" "What can be done to reduce the formaldehyde level?" (Online), Available: http://www.health.state.mm.us/divs/eh/indoorair/voc/formaldehyde.htm

USEFUL WEBSITES

"About Mold and Dampness," (Online), Available: http://www.cal-iaq.org/mold/about-mold

Allergy and Environmental Sensitivity Support and Research Association, AESSRA, 2008 *Chemical sensitivity and MCS*, (Online), Available: www.aessra.org/chemical-sensitivity-and-mcs.php

American College of Toxicology, 2012 *International Journal of Toxicology*, "Final Report on the Safety Assessment of Sodium Lauryl Sulfate and Ammonium Lauryl Sulfate," 2006 (Online), Available: ijt.sagepub.com/content/2/7/127

Antol, Marie Nadine 1996, Book, *Healing Teas*, "A Practical Guide to the Medicinal Teas of the World – From Chamomile to Garlic, From Essiac to Kombucha," "How to Prepare and Use Teas to Maximize Your Health," (Online), Available: www.amazon.com/

Bijlsma, Nicole 2010, *Healthy Home Healthy* Family, "Chemicals, Chemicals Everywhere!" Pg 241- 2 Available: www.aces.edu.au

Birnbaum, Linda S. and Staskal, Daniele F. 2004, 'Brominated flame retardants: cause for concern?' *Environmental Health Perspectives*, vol. 112, no. 1, pp. 9-17 (Online), Available: www.ncbi.nlm.nih.gov/.../v.112(1); Jan 2004

Boudewijn Gregory, *How Does a Volt Stick Work?* (Online), Available: www.eHow.co.uk/voltstick

Bridges Betty, n.d. *Practical Asthma Reviews, Fragrances and Chemical Sensitivities,*

(Online), Available: www.ameliaww.com/fpin/fpin.htm

Bremness, Lesley 1988, *The Complete Book of Herbs*, pg 213 "Basic Herbal Preparations," Book, ISBN 0 86438 066 6, © Dorling Kindersley Limited, 9 Henrietta Street, London WC2E 8PS, Reprinted 1991, 1992. (Online), Available: www.amazon.com/

California Department of Public Health, 2011, Indoor Air Quality Program, *A Brief Guide to Mold, Moisture, and Your Home*, "Mold Basics," (Online), Available: http://www.epa.gov/mold/moldbasics.html

Campbell, Giraud W., D.O. 1972, in association with Robert B. Stone, *A Doctor's Proven New Home Cure for Arthritis*, published by Thorsons Publishers Limited, Wellingborough, Northamptonshire NN8 2RQ, England, ISBN 0-7225-1911-7

Clotfelter, Susan n.d., Book, *The Herb Tea Book*, "Blending, Brewing and Savoring Teas for Every Meal and Occasion," (Online), Available: at time of writing, www.amazon.com/

Dewey David Lawrence, 1999 *Food For Thought, Colognes – Perfumes – Pesticides, Are They Slowly Killing You?* (Online), Available: www.dldewey.com/perfume.htm

Dunne, Lavon J., Book, *Nutrition Almanac*, Nutrition Search, Inc. Kirschmann, John D. Director, (Online), Available: www.amazon.com/

Dust Mite Information Centre, 2004, (Online), Available: http://www.com/findmites.htm

dust-mite.net, 2012 (Online), Available: http://www.dust-mite.net/dust-mite-control/

GEOMANCY

Further reading:

www.britishdowsers.org

www.canadiandowsers.org

www.dulwichhealth.co.uk

www.rolfgordon.co.uk

www.fengshuisociety.org.uk

www.geomancygroup.org

Grant, Lucinda 1997, "Electrical Sensitivity as an Emerging Illness," (Online), Available: http://www.tldp.com/issue/179/emf179.htm

Health Risks of Perfume, April 2002 (Online), Available: www.ourlittleplace.com

Hopman, Ellen Evert 1995, Book, *A Druid's Herbal for the Sacred Earth Year*, (Online), Available: www.amazon.com/

Indoor Quality Program, Sep 3, 2014, "Mold and Dampness," (Online), Available: www.cdph.ca.gov>Hone>Programs>Section

Kramer Shelley R., n.d. (Online), Available: www.healthy-communications.com/slsmostdangerousirritant.html

Lorber, M 2007, 'Exposure of Americans to polybrominated diphenyl ethers,' *Journal of Exposure Science and Environmental Epidemiology*, vol. 18 (Online), Available: www.mendeley.com/.../exposure-americans-polybromin...-United States

Mahan & Escott-Stump, 1996, Book, *Krause's Food, Nutrition & Diet*, (Online), Available: www.amazon.com/

Marcin, Marietta Marshall 1999, *Herbal Tea Gardens*, "22 Plans for your

Enjoyment and Well-Being," (Online), Available: www.amazon.com/

Minnesota Department of Health, June 2012, *Mold and Moisture in Homes*, "What are the health concerns?" "Are the risks greater for some people?" "Are some molds more hazardous than others?" "Home Investigation," "Should I test for mold?" Mold Clean-up and Removal," (Online), Available: http://www.health.state.mn.us/divs/eh/indoorair/mold/index/htm;

"Mold Cleanup Guidelines," (Online), Available: http://www.epa.gov/mold/cleanupguidelines.html

National Cancer Institute, 2011, "Formaldehyde," (Online), Available: www.cancer.org>...>Other Carcinogens>In the Workplace

NCRP Scientific Committee, 1995, 89-3: "Draft Report on Extremely Low Frequency Electric and Magnetic Fields, July/August 1995, p.12-15. (Online), Available: http://www.equilibrauk.com/emfsbio.shtml

Occupational Health and Safety Unit, March 2010, University of Queensland Australia, *Organic solvents guideline*, "Common Causes of Organic Solvents", (Online), Available: www.uq.edu.au/ohs/pdfs/organicsolvents.pdf

Powerwatch Appliances Factsheet 2012, (Online), Available: www.powerwatch.org.uk/elf/appliances.asp

Reed Gibson PhD Pamela, 2003, *An Introduction to Multiple Chemical Sensitivity and Electrical Sensitivity*, James Madison University, The Environmental Illness Resource (Online), Available:

www.ei-resources.org/.../multiple-chemical-sensitivity.../an-intro

Russell, 2001, *Fragrance Sensitivity*, 2001 (Online), Available: allnaturalbeauty.us/chemicalsensitivities

Chemical Sensitivities and Perfume, Chemicals and Pesticides, (Online), Available: allnaturalbeauty.us/chemicalsensitivities, then http://jrussellshealth.org

Rutherford, Theresa 2011, *Compost Happens*, Online, www.aaee.org.au/

docs/.../Non-Toxic%20Cleanin%20Workshop.pdf

Shekut, Sue 2009, (Online), Available: workingwellresources.com/.../nasas-top-ten-plants-to-remove-formal...

Stebbins, Kathleen 2011, "Allergic Reactions", (Online), Available: *The Allergy Site* http://livestrong.com/article/159171-the-disadvantages-of-sodium-laureth-sulfate/

Stratham Bill, 2002 *The Chemical Maze 2nd Edition*, "Your Guide to Food Additives and Cosmetic Ingredients," pp. 117, 107 Available: possibility.com.au/

U.S. House of Representatives, 1986, "*Neurotoxins: At Home and the Workplace*," Report by the Committee on Science & Technology, Sept. 16, 1986, (Report 99-827), (Online), Available: www.herc.org/news/perfume/scents.htm

Vance Judi, 1998 Alkalize for Health, 2000 *Toxic Cosmetic Ingredient List*, (Online), Available: www.alkalizeforhealth.net/Ltoxiccosmetics.htm

Vegan Peace, 2004 (Online), Available: www.veganpeace.com/ingredients.htm

Virtue, Doreen Ph.D., Spiritual doctor of psychology (Online), Available: www.AngelTherapy.com

Yvonne, 2010 *Plants Absorb Indoor Pollution* Online, www.earthwitchery.com/pollution.html

Ziem, Grace M.D. 2001, *Chemical Awareness*, "Why Scents Don't Make Sense," (Online), Available: http://www.ecoviva.com/html/synthetic-fragrances.html

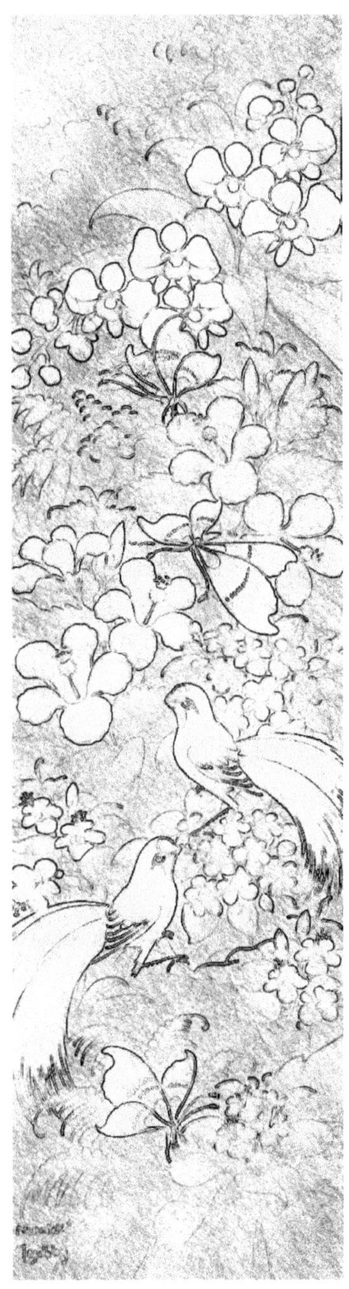

"Murniati" by Tegallalang, Iwayan Arnaya, Bali

Index

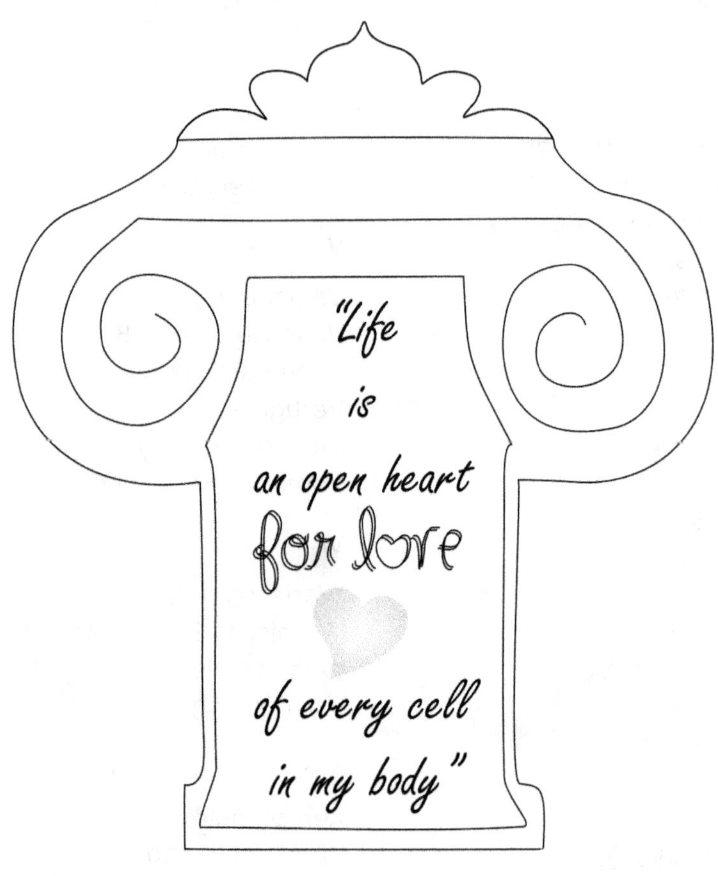
"Life
is
an open heart
for love
of every cell
in my body"

RECOMMENDATIONS

Rainwater

RAINFOREST DEW™, 100% Rainwater

Oxygenated, ultra-finely filtered, with a molecular structure that allows full absorption of oxygen, therefore hydration can contribute to an environment primarily desirable for physical wellbeing, creating an inner glow.

10 Litres - with tap for easy access - in-house, groups, on-sites, bench tops

1.5L - table & travel

600mL - goes everywhere

600mL with SPORT cap - for hand free opening

350 mL with SPORT cap

350mL - thirst quencher

Available:

Paradise Waters Pty Ltd

Web: www.rainforestdewonline.com

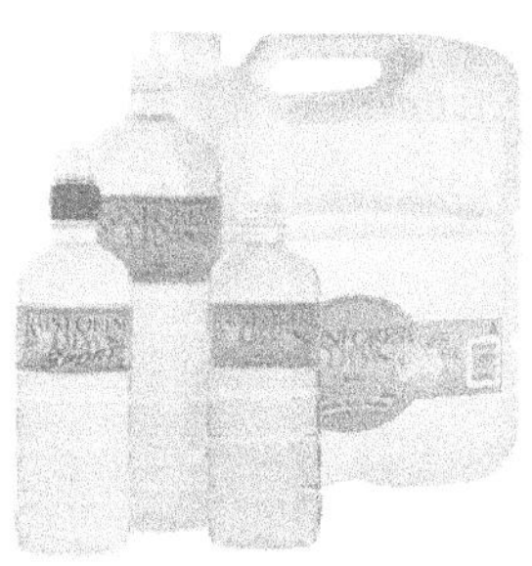

Natural Cleaning Aids

Available:

Abode

Website: www.buildingbiology.com.au

Music for All Occasions

Available:

Lifestyle Music

"Nature, Meditation, Health & Wellbeing, Classical, Spa"

Website: www.lifestylemusic.com.au

Accommodation

Available:

Exclusive Retreats

Misty Mountains Eco Stay

Website: www.romanticretreats.com.au Click on Misty Mountain

The Best from the Library of Nancy F. Hegarty/Newitt

CDs

DAILY RELAXATION MEDITATION

For re-energising, re-balancing and gentle healing this is a must if you are in the healing profession, feel overworked or simply feeling stuck in life. Rise from this session feeling the amazing benefits. This is not your average every day relaxation meditation. This new type of meditation enables you to stay focused.

PAIN MANAGEMENT & PREPARATION FOR HEALING

This meditation will create a healthy atmosphere within you and around you. If you are willing to accept new positive thoughts healing can happen.

MEDITATION FOR MUSTERING INTENSIVE ENERGY

Feel the power as you draw upon the 12th Chakra Universal Cosmic Energy while in a higher state of consciousness that allows you to expand beyond any limitations in your life.

AN INTRODUCTION TO A HEALTHY LIFE

The Most Loving 286 Life Affirmations, the Gift to Creating Miracles is easy listening at home and play, going to and from work. Experience the freedom as you create an even more enjoyable life.

EBooks

THE AUSTRALIAN MASSAGE ... Feeling the Healing

Practical movements for the beginner

Enhancing skills for the experienced practitioner

Professional instructions with many intricate, close-up photographs

Originally produced for students at Australian colleges

SIMPLE FOODS TO HEAL YOUR BODY

Recommended for permanent healing guidance

Shows delicious healing foods for ailments A to Z

Keep this instant guide with you when shopping for food if you have any ailment; look up the ailment that is listed from A to Z, choose the foods that you like to commence the healing process and enjoy eating your way to better health; also includes a hint of Metaphysics and an introduction to Modern and Traditional Feng Shui.

THE AUSTRALIAN ADVANCED AND METAPHYSICAL MASSAGE

Includes Proprioceptive Neuromuscular Facilitation Stretches (PNFs) to the Neck and Spine, Sciatic Release, Freeing the Shoulders, Releasing Knotted Muscles, Palm Release, Chopping and Pummelling Major Muscles, Shoulder, Elbow and Wrist Stretches, Hip, Knee and Ankle Stretches, Pre-Sports and Post Sports Massage, Pregnant Lady Massage Techniques, Hot Herbal Towel Applications, Metaphysics and the Body, Invigorating Affirmations for Re-Aligning Vertebrae and Spiritual Advancement. This expands in-depth appreciation for the basically trained beginner, and broadens the professional practitioner's experiences; also includes an introduction to Kinesiology, Lymphatic Massage and Reflexology.

BOOKs

THE AUSTRALIAN MASSAGE - Feeling the Healing

Practical movements for the beginner

Enhancing skills for the experienced practitioner

Professional instructions with many intricate, close-up photographs

Originally produced for students at Australian colleges

SIMPLE FOODS TO HEAL YOUR BODY

Recommended for permanent healing guidance

Shows delicious healing foods for ailments A to Z

Keep this instant guide with you when shopping for food if you have any ailment; look up the ailment that is listed from A to Z, choose the foods that you like to commence the healing process and enjoy eating your way to better health; also includes a hint of Metaphysics and an introduction to Modern and Traditional Feng Shui.

THE AUSTRALIAN ADVANCED AND METAPHYSICAL MASSAGE

includes Proprioceptive Neuromuscular Facilitation Stretches (PNFs) to the Neck and Spine, Sciatic Release, Freeing the Shoulders, Releasing Knotted Muscles, Palm Release, Chopping and Pummelling Major Muscles, Shoulder, Elbow and Wrist Stretches, Hip, Knee and Ankle Stretches, Pre-Sports and Post Sports Massage, Pregnant Lady Massage Techniques, Hot Herbal Towel Applications, Metaphysics and the Body, Invigorating Affirmations for Re-Aligning Vertebrae and Spiritual Advancement. This expands in-depth appreciation for the basically trained beginner, and broadens the professional practitioner's experiences; includes an introduction to Kinesiology, Lymphatic Massage and Reflexology.

DVD

THE AUSTRALIAN MASSAGE

Professional instructions with detailed practical movements for the beginner, and enhancing skills for the qualified practitioner, showing how to perform the complete sequence with no stops from commencement to finish.

Pain Management & Preparation for Healing

PAIN MANAGEMENT & PREPARATION FOR HEALING

THIS MEDITATION WILL CREATE A HEALTHY ATMOSPHERE BOTH WITHIN YOU & AROUND YOU

Healing can happen!

Being pain free and totally synchronized with life is your Divine Right now. Listening and following this meditation has the power to prepare your body for healing and can create miracles in your life. *Pain Management & Preparation for Healing* is easy to follow enabling you to go within, connect with that part of you that knows how to heal and where you know pure love. Knowing each body cell has Divine intelligence, you listen to what it tells you and know that its advice is valid. You are always safe, protected and guided as you feel how your body wants to be healed.

Daily Relaxation Meditation

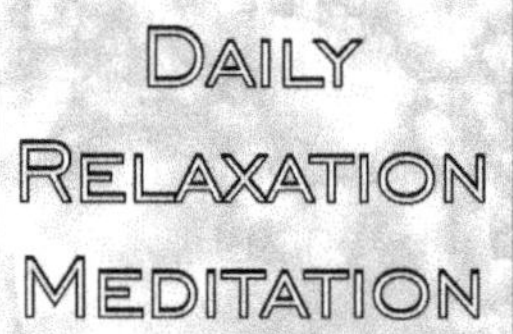

Meditation for Mustering Intensive Energy

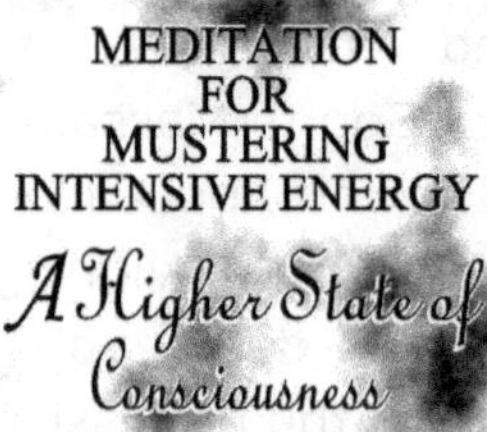

An Introduction to a Healthy Life

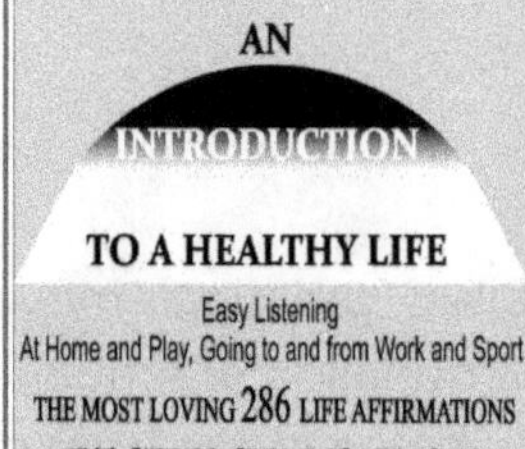

Available: *www.paradisewaters1.com*

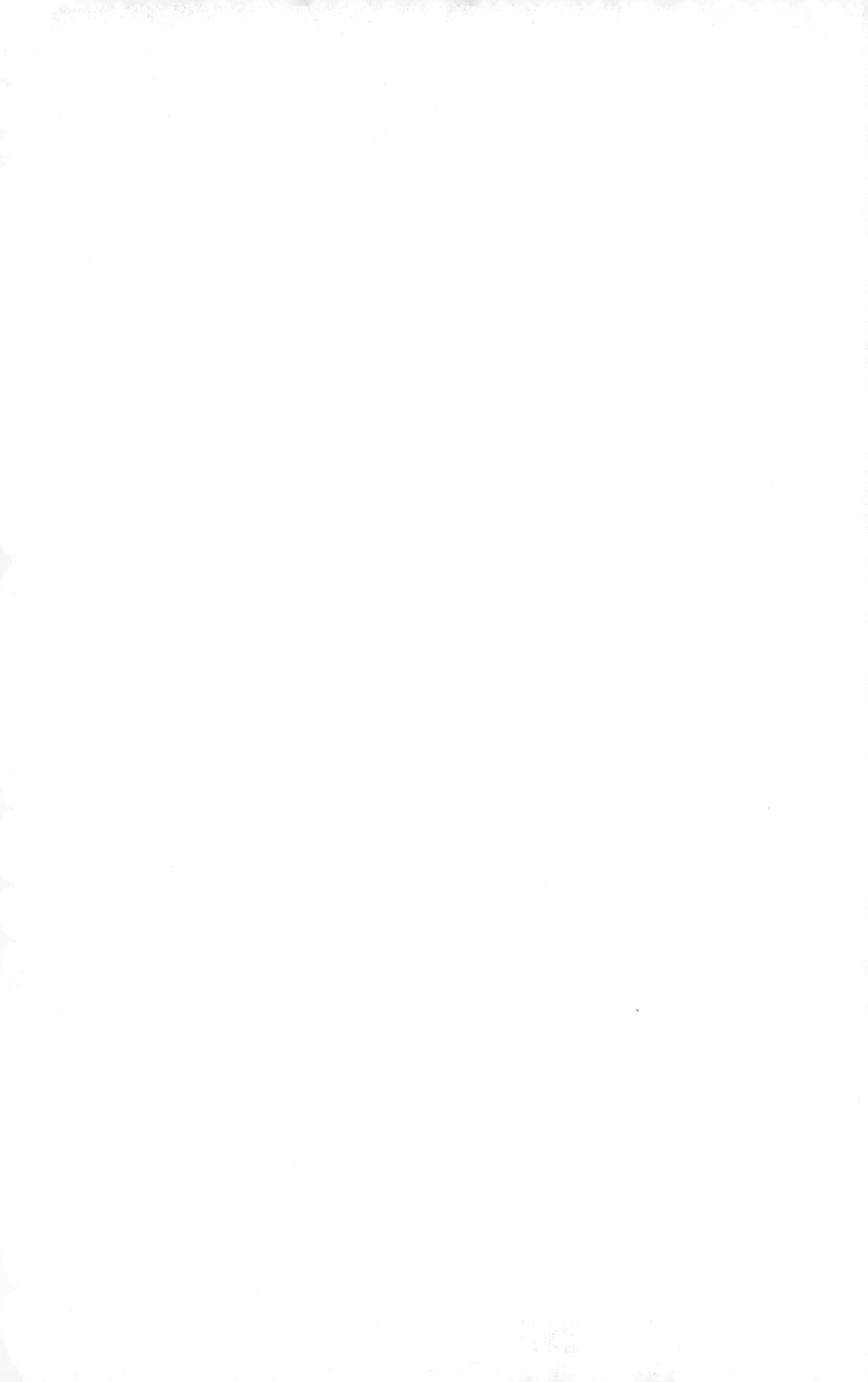

www.ingramcontent.com/pod-product-compliance
Lightning Source LLC
Chambersburg PA
CBHW072143020426
42334CB00018B/1870

* 9 7 8 0 9 9 2 4 0 3 4 7 8 *